Madhavan G. Nair
05/09/1993

INNOVATIONS IN UROLOGIC ONCOLOGY

INNOVATIONS IN UROLOGIC ONCOLOGY

Selected Papers from a Northwestern University
Cancer Center Symposium
in Honor of
John T. Grayhack, M.D.

Edited by
Steven Rosen, M.D.
Chung Lee, Ph.D.
Martin S. Tallman, M.D.

Northwestern University Cancer Center

Precept Press, Inc., Chicago

Library of Congress Catalog Card Number: 91-67426

International Standard Book Number: 0-944496-25-3

96 95 94 93 92 5 4 3 2 1

Composition by Interface Studio, Inc., Northbrook, IL

Printed in the United States of America

CONTENTS

SECTION III – BLADDER CANCER

SECTION IV–TESTIS CANCER

PREFACE

THE MATERIALS ASSEMBLED IN these pages grew out of the Malnati Symposium on Innovations in Cancer Diagnosis and Treatment, held October 4-5, 1990, in Chicago under the sponsorship of the Northwestern Unversity Cancer Center of the McGaw Medical Center of Northwestern University. The symposium was the first of an annual series of educational events made possible by a gift to the cancer center from the Malnati family of Chicago. The symposia will be coordinated by the Office of Continuing Education of the Northwestern University School of Medicine.

The objectives of this and future Malnati symposia are to provide state-of-the-art information on cancer research, diagnosis, and treatment. Programs will be designed to appeal not only to medical oncologists but also to internists, surgeons, hematologists, microbiologists, and other medical specialists interested in the most recent developments in oncology.

The subject of urologic oncology was chosen for the inaugural symposium in honor of John T. Grayhack, M.D., an internationally known authority on urologic oncology, who retired at the end of 1990 as chairman of the Department of Urology of the Northwestern University School of Medicine. Dr. Grayhack also participated in the program as Distinguished Professor Lecturer.

As will also be true in the future, a core faculty made up of faculty members of the Northwestern University School of Medicine was joined by guest faculty from other medical schools and teaching institutions in this country and abroad in conducting the 1990 symposium.

It was the hope in gathering together these symposium materials and preparing them for wider distribution in permanent form that the educational benefits accruing to the attendees could in this way be at least partially shared with oncologists and other medical specialists throughout the country.

CONTRIBUTORS/FACULTY MEMBERS

R. BIHRLE, M.D., Associate Professor, Department of Urology, Indiana University Medical Center, Indianapolis, Indiana

WILLIAM CATALONA, M.D., Professor and Chairman, Department of Surgery, Division of Urologic Surgery, Washington University Medical School, St. Louis, Missouri

SUSAN COHN, M.D., Assistant Professor of Pediatrics, Northwestern University Medical School; Division of Hematology/Oncology, Children's Memorial Hospital, Chicago, Illinois

E. DAVID CRAWFORD, M.D., Professor and Chairman, Division of Urology, University of Colorado Health Science Center, Denver, Colorado

TRACY CURLEY, R.N., Genitourinary Oncology Service, Division of Solid Tumor Oncology, Department of Medicine, Memorial Sloan-Kettering Cancer Center, New York City, New York

JOHN P. DONOHUE, M.D., Distinguished Professor and Chairman, Department of Urology, Indiana University Hospital, Indiana University Medical Center, Indianapolis, Indiana

CHAU-JYE FONG, M.D., Graduate Student, Departments of Pathology and Urology, Northwestern University Medical School, Chicago, Illinois

R. S. FOSTER, M.D., Assistant Professor, Department of Urology, Indiana University Medical Center, Indianapolis, Indiana

JOHN T. GRAYHACK, M.D., Professor and Chairman, Department of Urology, Northwestern University Medical School, Chicago, Illinois

KIYOSHI ITO, M.D., Ben May Institute and Department of Biochemistry and Molecular Biology, University of Chicago, Chicago, Illinois

JACQUELINE M. IVERSEN, R.Ph., Genitourinary Oncology Service, Division of Solid Tumor Oncology, Department of Medicine, Memorial Sloan-Kettering Cancer Center, New York City, New York

MERRILL KIES, M.D., Associate Professor of Medicine, Section of Hematology/Oncology, Northwestern University Medical School, Chicago, Illinois

JOHN KOKONTIS, M.D., Ben May Institute and Department of Biochemistry and Molecular Biology, University of Chicago, Chicago, Illinois

JAMES KOZLOWSKI, M.D., Associate Professor of Urology, Surgery, and Tumor Cell Biology; Director, Genitourinary Oncology Program, Northwestern University Medical School, Chicago, Illinois

CHUNG LEE, Ph.D., Professor of Urology; Professor of Cell, Molecular, and Structural Biology; Director of Urology Research laboratories, Northwestern University Medical School, Chicago, Illinois

SHUTSUNG LIAO, Ph.D., Professor of Biochemistry and Molecular Biology, Ben May Institute and Department of Biochemistry and Molecular Biology, University of Chicago, Chicago, Illinois

W. MARSTEN LINEHAN, M.D., Head, Urologic Oncology Section, Surgery Branch, National Cancer Institute, Bethesda, Maryland

XIANGLIN LIU, M.D., Research Associate, Department of Urology, Northwestern University Medical School, Chicago, Illinois

MICHAEL T. LOTZE, M.D., Visiting Professor, Department of Surgery, and Associate Director, Pittsburgh Cancer Institute, Pittsburgh, Pennsylvania

CRAIG R. NICHOLS, M.D., Assistant Professor of Medicine, Division of Hematology/Oncology, Indiana University Medical Center, Indianapolis, Indiana

ANDREW NOVICK, M.D., Chairman, Department of Urology, Cleveland Clinic, Cleveland, Ohio

RYIOCHI OYASU, M.D., Professor of Pathology and Urology, Northwestern University Medical School, Chicago, Illinois

JOHN RAFFENSPERGER, M.D., Professor of Pediatrics, Department of Pediatrics, Children's Memorial Hospital, Chicago, Illinois

MARTIN RESNICK, M.D., Lester Persky Professor and Chief, Department of Urology, Case Western Reserve University School of Medicine, Cleveland, Ohio

STEVEN ROSEN, M.D., Professor of Medicine, Section of Hematology/Oncology; Director, Northwestern University Cancer Center, Chicago, Illinois

RANDALL G. ROWLAND, M.D., Ph.D., Professor of Urology, Indiana University School of Medicine, Indianapolis, Indiana

PETER T. SCARDINO, M.D., Professor and Chairman, Scott Department of Urology, Baylor College of Medicine, Houston, Texas

HOWARD SCHER, M.D., Assistant Attending Physician, Genitourniary Service, Division of Solid Tumor Oncology, Department of Medicine, Memorial Sloan-Kettering Cancer Center, New York City, New York

EDWARD R. SHERWOOD, Ph.D., Postdoctorate Fellow and Research Associate, Department of Urology and Cancer Center, Northwestern University Medical School, Chicago, Illinois

RAMANANDA SHETTY, M.D., Assistant Professor of Radiology, Division of Radiation Oncology, Northwestern University Medical School, Chicago, Illinois

BRYAN P. SHUMAKER, M.D., Director, Laser Center, St. Joseph Mercy Hospital, Pontiac, Michigan; Adjutant Assistant Professor of Physics, Oakland University, Rochester, Michigan

MARK SOLOWAY, M.D., Professor and Chief, Urologic Oncology, University of Tennessee, Memphis, Tennessee

DEBRA M. SUTKOWSKI, Graduate Student, Tumor Cell Biology Program, Department of Urology, Northwestern University Medical School, Chicago, Illinois

MARTIN S. TALLMAN, M.D., Assistant Professor of Medicine, Section of Hematology/Oncology, Northwestern University Medical School, Chicago, Illinois

J. A. THORNHILL, M. Ch., F.R.C.S.I., Urologic Fellow, Department of Urology, Indiana University Medical Center, Indianapolis, Indiana

WILLIAM TONG, Ph.D., Program of Molecular Pharmacology and Therapeutics, Memorial Sloan-Kettering Cancer Center, New York City, New York

ROBERT P. WEAVER, M.D., Scott Department of Urology, Baylor College of Medicine, Houston, Texas

ALAN YAGODA, M.D., Professor of Clinical Medicine, New York Hospital-Cornell University Medical Center, New York City, New York

1

RECEPTORS AND MOLECULAR ACTIONS OF ANDROGENS

Shutsung Liao, Ph.D.; Kiyoshi Ito, M.D.; and John Kokontis, M.D.

Differential Functions of Testosterone and 5α-Dihydrotestosterone

MANY STEROID HORMONES ENTER target cells and bind to steroid receptors (SRs) without metabolic conversion. However, in the prostate and many other target organs of androgens, testosterone (T), the major testicular androgen circulating in blood, acts mainly after its conversion to 5α-dihydrotestosterone (DHT) by a 3-keto 5α steroid reductase (5α-reductase) in the target cells. DHT then forms a complex with a specific receptor that interacts with a nuclear acceptor site presumably containing DNA with an androgen response element (ARE) and other factors important for the regulation of gene transcription. Certain aspects of embryonic male urogenital tract differentiation, growth of kidney and muscle, testicular functions, and sexual behavior appear to utilize T, whereas DHT is the active form of androgens in many peripheral androgen-sensitive tissues. Both T and DHT appear to function by binding to ARs coded by the same AR gene, but the 2 androgens appear to act differently. The precise reason for this difference has not been clearly identified, but the following factors may be important:

1. The local concentrations and metabolic conversion of T and DHT in different target cells are different.

The work described in this article was supported by Grants DK 37694 and DK 41670 from the National Institutes of Health.

2. T binds to AR less firmly than DHT, because T dissociates more rapidly than DHT from AR.

3. The conformations of the T-R and DHT-R complexes may be different.

4. The transactivation of genes in different cells may have different requirements for the level and replenishment of androgen-receptor complexes.

5. Other transcription factors or oncoproteins may interact with T-R and DHT-R complexes differently.

Although as much as 20% of the total androgens in human blood is DHT, DHT produced by 5α-reductase in the target cells appears to be more effective in promoting transactivation of target genes than the circulating DHT. Among some of the possible explanations are that (1) DHT bound to blood proteins may not be as effective as the endogenous DHT, and (2) intracellular localization of 5α-reductase, DHT-metabolizing enzymes, and AR may favor the utilization of newly produced DHT over the external DHT.

Structure and Inhibitors of 5α-Reductase

Understanding the differences in the ways T and DHT act in androgen-sensitive organs and the structure and the mechanism involved in regulation of 5α-reductase are important for the design of new compounds that may have a chemotherapeutic value in the control of the abnormal growth of prostates and androgen-sensitive tumors. Excessive formation and/or retention of DHT in target cells have been implicated in certain androgen-dependent pathological conditions, including benign prostatic hyperplasia (BPH), acne, male-pattern baldness, and female idiopathic hirsutism. Therefore, appropriate 5α-reductase inhibitors (figure 1-1) should be very useful in selective treatment of these DHT-dependent abnormalities without affecting T-dependent androgen-sensitive organs. The primary structure of 5α-reductases, elucidated from cDNA sequences, also can provide new information essential in analyzing reductase gene regulation, mutations, intracellular membrane localization, and

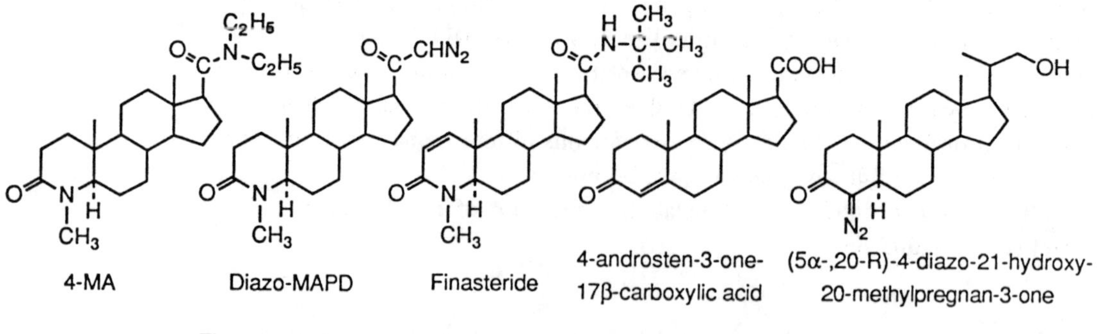

Figure 1-1. Representative 5α-reductase inhibitors.

dynamics of the reductase at the molecular level. The reductase activity may be regulated by cellular substances (including lipid components) that interact with the hydrophobic enzyme and/or affect the membrane localization of the reductase. Polyclonal and monoclonal antibodies, as well as various nucleotide probes for 5α-reductase, can be useful in basic studies as well as in diagnostic analysis of 5α-reductase-linked abnormalities.

Androgen Receptor Binding of Androgens and Antiandrogens

The structural requirements for biological function and binding of steroids to the AR suggest that multiple sites of an androgenic steroid are bound by the AR as if the steroid molecule was being enveloped. This is in marked contrast to steroid-metabolizing enzymes, antisteroid antibodies, or blood steroid-binding proteins, which generally recognize only a portion of the steroid molecule. Antisteroid antibodies can effectively remove steroids peripherally attached to these nonreceptor steroid-binding proteins but not those bound to their SRs. The concept of "steroid enveloping by SR" implies that a steroid hormone can substantially alter the conformation of its receptor protein, especially at the hormone-binding domain.

Classical steroidal antiandrogens (figure 1-2), such as cyproterone and its 17α-acetate, appear to act by competing with androgens for binding to AR. Flutamide, a nonsteroidal antiandrogen, was found to act in vivo by the same mechanism, apparently after a conversion to hydroxyflutamide. Anandron, on the other hand, appeared

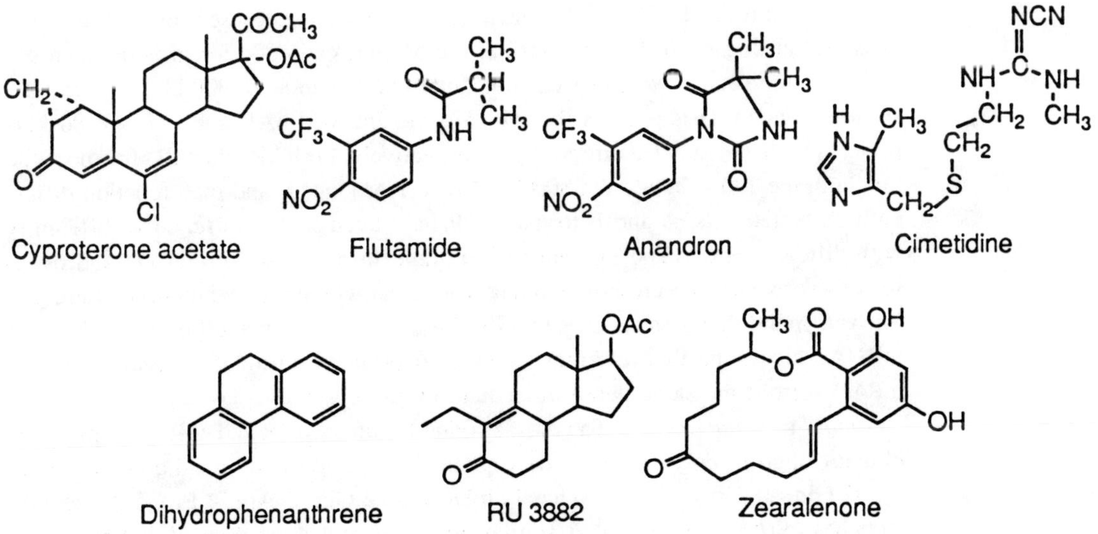

Figure 1-2. Representative antiandrogens.

to act directly by binding to AR. Many antiandrogens bind to AR with a low affinity (usually much less than 1/50th of natural androgens), but they are useful as chemotherapeutic agents because they do not show significant side effects or toxicity.

Small compounds that can easily enter the androgen-binding cavity of AR (a high rate of association) and are trapped inside the binding cavity (a low rate of dissociation) may act as antiandrogens. Phenanthrene, a conjugated flat molecule that could presumably associate rapidly with AR, has a low affinity toward AR. In contrast, 9,10-dihydrophenanthrene, a compound having greater structural flexibility that may allow the 2 end rings to conform to a structure compatible with the binding cavity of AR, has 80-fold higher affinity than phenanthrene toward AR. In castrated rats, 9,10-dihydrophenanthrene can reduce the androgen-dependent growth of the ventral prostate, seminal vesicle, and coagulating gland, whereas phenanthrene is essentially inactive as an antiandrogen.

Studies with antiandrogens have clearly indicated that the antagonistic activity is associated with a physical blockage of receptor binding to androgens, and that binding of these antiandrogens does not require the presence of specific functional groups. However, the functional (17β-hydroxyl and 3-keto) groups may provide a high affinity binding of androgens or antiandrogens to ARs.

Structures and Functions of Androgen Receptors

Overall structure. Cloning and sequencing of the cDNA and determination of the deduced amino acid sequences of ARs have made it possible to analyze the roles of different AR domains in eliciting androgenic responses. Based on our nucleotide sequence analysis of AR cDNAs, the open reading frames present in hAR and rAR cDNAs, starting from the first ATG at the 5′ end, can code for proteins with 918 and 902 amino acids, which have a molecular mass of about 97-100 kDa (figure 1-3). If the second ATG is used as the initiator, the encoded hAR and rAR are 80 kDa proteins with 734 and 733 amino acids, respectively, for hAR and rAR. It is possible that both the 100 kDa and the 80 kDa ARs are produced, and they function differently in target cells. A and B forms of PR have been shown to function differently with different HRE. The existence of multiple forms of AR in normal androgen-sensitive organs has been shown, but it is not clear whether they function differently. We have found that prostate cancer cells (LNCaP) can produce different sizes of AR mRNA, suggesting that different forms of ARs may be produced from their own mRNAs (from the same gene) other than by proteolysis.

Amino-terminal domain. The most striking feature of hAR and rAR is the presence of many oligo-or poly (amino acid) sequences in the amino terminal domain. There are 17 Gln, 27 Gly, 8 Pro stretches in hAR and 22 Gln, 5 Arg, 4 Pro, 5 Ala, 5 Gly stretches in rAR (figure 1-3). A similar but not identical amino acid motif recently was found for mouse AR. The Gln stretches are found in ARs from humans, rats,

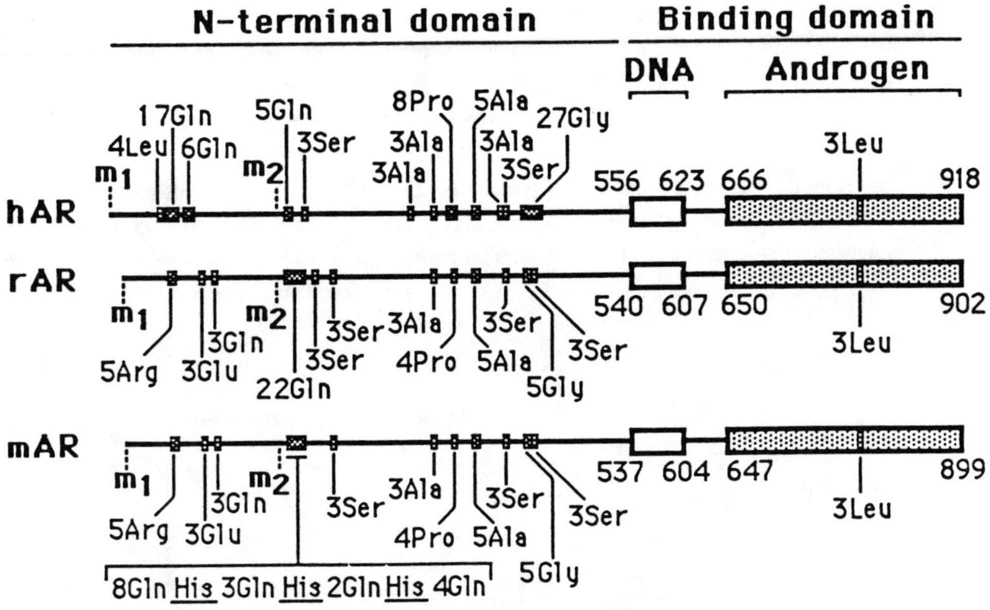

Figure 1-3. Amino acid sequences of ARs from human (h), rat (r) and mouse (m). The first and second methionines in the N-terminal domains are indicated by m_1 and m_2. The positions and the number of amino acids in each oligo- or poly (amino acid) are shown. The amino acid positions of the DNA- and androgen-binding domains are indicated by amino acid numbers started from m1.

and mice, but their distribution patterns are different. In mouse (m) AR, poly (Gln) is present as a discontinuous repeat of 8, 3, 2, and 4 Gln, with 1 His separating each group. Deletion or replacement of some of these sequences may show unusual changes in AR function and recycling patterns. Many regulatory gene products are known to contain poly (amino acid) sequences. Poly (Gly) and poly (Glu) are present in several homeotic genes. There is a Gln-stretch in rGR and a Glu-stretch in chicken progesterone receptor, but a long polyamino acid stretch is not present in other SRs. Therefore, some of the polyamino acid-recognizing factors may be species- and AR-specific and are unique to the regulation of the function and recycling of AR.

DNA- and androgen-binding domains. The amino acid sequences in the DNA-binding and androgen binding domains (excluding the hinge region between the 2 domains) are 100% identical among hAR, rAR, and mAR, and only 1 amino acid change (Gly to Ala in the first zinc finger region of the DNA-binding domain) in frog AR. This indicates that the transactivation functions in these domains recognize the same ARE and act by the same mechanism. The 68-amino acid cysteine-rich DNA-binding domains in hAR and rAR have an identical amino acid sequence, although there are 14 nucleotide changes. There is a high homology (75-80%) among

ARs and hPR, hGR, hMR in this DNA-binding domain. AR, GR, and PR also recognize the same HRE. The 253 amino acid sequence of the androgen-binding domain at the C-terminal end of hAR and rAR are identical, although there are 54 nucleotide differences in the DNA coding for this region. The homology in this domain among ARs, GR, PR, and MR is only 50-54%. However, 4 short regions within this domain have 65-100% sequence similarity among these receptors.

Although it has not been experimentally proven, the androgen-binding domain may have a region that may function as a transcription inhibitory component (figure 1-4), as has been suggested for other SRs and some nuclear hormone receptors. This

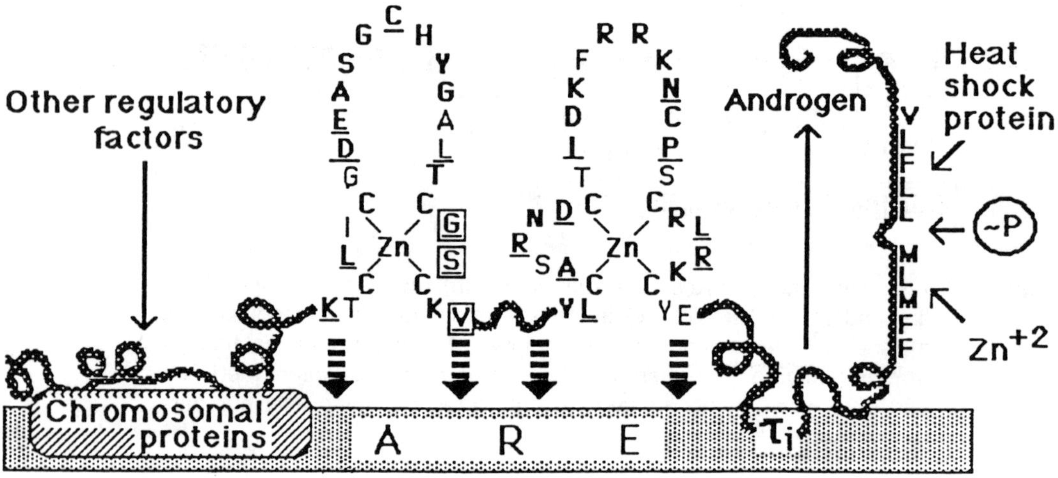

Figure 1-4. A hypothetical model indicating the roles of AR domains.

domain may inhibit the interaction of the DNA-binding domain with ARE. Binding of androgen to the domain may result in the removal of this interference. In the androgen-binding domain, at least 9 amino acid heptads contain Leu or other hydrophobic amino acids (e.g., Met, Phe, Val) at positions 1 and 8. These repeats may behave like a leucine zipper motif and provide a site for dimerization of ARs or AR and other transcription factors or oncoproteins. Homo- or hetero-dimerization of SRs or other transcriptional factors may play a key role in promoting positive or negative regulation of gene transcription.

Transactivation of a reporter gene. We have studied the activity of various transfected AR genes to transactivate a reporter gene. In the vector, pSG5-AR, the AR gene (cDNA) is linked to the SV40 early promotor, and a SV40 poly (A) signal is downstream of the AR gene. The reporter gene, chloramphenicol acetyl transferase (CAT) was linked downstream of the mouse mammary tumor virus (MMTV) long terminal repeat (LTR). The LTR segment contains a HRE that is recognized by GR as well as PR or AR. When androgen-insensitive and AR-deficient human prostate cancer cells (PC-3) were transfected with pSG5-AR, the cells produced a large quantity of AR. Treatment of PC-3 cells with androgens after cotransfection with pSG5-AR and MMTV-CAT stimulated CAT gene expression. The AR-dependent transactivation of CAT gene was inhibited by antiandrogen (hydroxyflutamide).

Regulation of AR gene expression in the prostate and various cells. Using a nick-translated fragment of AR-cDNA as a probe and Northern blot analysis, we analyzed the level of AR mRNA in many male and female organs and normal, hyperplastic, and cancerous human prostate (clinical specimens and established prostatic cancer cells, such as LNCaP and PC3 cells). In rat prostate, androgens appear to autoregulate AR mRNA. Androgen repression of the steady-state level of its receptor mRNA was also observed by other investigators. A study carried out by Sanborn in collaboration with our group showed that the AR-mRNA (9.5 kb) level increased 5-fold in Sertoli cells and peritubular cells after hypophysectomy of rats. This effect was reversed after the hypophysectomized rats were treated with testosterone. FSH, in vitro, increased AR-mRNA up to 5-fold in Sertoli cells but not in peritubular cells.

Structure and Mutations of Androgen Receptor Gene, Androgen Insensitivity, and Abnormality in Steroid Responses

The AR gene has been localized to the q11–q12 region of the human X-chromosome. The total length of the hAR gene appears to be >90 kb and the AR coding region was separated over 8 exons. There are striking similarities in the intron-exon organization among the SR genes. AR and other SRs are each encoded by a single-copy gene located on separate chromosomes (retinoic acid and thyroid hormone receptors seemed to have at least 2 genes on different chromosomes). All exon-intron junctions in hAR, hER, and cPR are located at similar positions, although the lengths of the introns are quite different.

Abnormalities in the responses to androgens have been observed in man and other animals, and have involved target organs as well as tumors. Androgen insensitivity can be caused by a mutation or abnormal expression of the genes for the AR or 5α-reductase, or defects in other cellular components that are needed to exert normal androgen responses in AR- and 5α-reductase-positive cells. A deficiency in 5α-reductase has been related to abnormal male sexual differentiation, whereas a defect in the X-chromosome-linked AR was considered to be responsible for syndromes of androgen resistance, such as testicular feminization (tfm). Mutations in AR genes have been observed in 15 individuals with abnormal androgen responses. So far, the abnormalities in AR genes are due to point mutations rather than gross structural alterations of the AR gene. Mutations in the androgen-binding domain have resulted in changes in 1 amino acid, introduction of a premature stop codon, deletion of part or all of a domain, or an alternative splicing. Many point mutations so far analyzed involved G to A mutations. It is known that the intracellular spontaneous deamination of 5-methylcystosine in DNA produces thymine, causing a GT-mismatch, which may be corrected by a repair pathway involving a GT-binding protein; if uncorrected, it may lead to a G to A transition during DNA replication.

We have also found that the AR gene in the androgen-sensitive prostate cancer cells, LNCaP, has a G to A mutation that changes amino acid 876 in the androgen-binding domain from Thr to Ala. The mutated AR was more efficient than normal AR in utilizing progesterone and 17β-estradiol as the hormonal ligand in the transactivation of a CAT gene (see above) cotransfected into the androgen-insensitive prostate cancer cells, PC-3. Surprisingly, hydroxyflutamide was also active in the CAT gene transactivation. Understanding of AR mutation, therefore, may be important in selecting appropriate hormones or antagonists for treatment of prostate cancers.

Intracellular Recycling of Androgen Receptors and Receptor Function

Dynamic status of prostate androgen receptors. The dynamic status of AR in prostate cells has been studied by incubation of rat ventral prostate with radioactive androgens in the presence and absence of respiratory poisons or inhibitors of protein and RNA synthesis, and also by isotope chasing of the radioactive A-R complexes. In the presence of 2,4-dinitrophenol, the AR is rapidly deactivated (half-life, 2 min) to an inactive form (R°) that does not bind androgen unless it is reactivated by an energy-dependent process to the androgen-binding form (R). A majority of the A-R complexes formed may not bind to DNA/chromatin unless they are "transformed" by a temperature-dependent process. It is not clear whether this is due to the need for a chemical modification of the A-R complexes or to the association/dissociation of other cellular factors such as a heat shock protein (figure 1-4). Isotope-chasing experiments with labeled androgen indicate that the steps involved in AR recycling between chromatin-bound and cytosolic forms are slow compared to other steps in the recycling process, and the A-R complex has a half-life of >50 min in this part of the cycle.

Androgen receptor recycling and post-transcriptional regulation. Although steroid hormones have significant effects on transcription of specific genes, the evidence is strong for post-transcriptional regulation of gene products by steroids. In many target cells or organs, steroid hormones increase the rate of the synthesis of mRNAs for specific proteins 2- to 5-fold but increase the cellular mRNA levels 20- to 50-fold. Steroid hormones, therefore, appear to alter the stability of induced mRNA in their target cells. More than 20 yr ago, we suggested that S-R complexes not only can bind DNA to promote specific gene transcription, but can also bind RNA and regulate processing, transport, stabilization, and/or utilization of RNA. Binding of various S-R complexes to RNA or ribonucleoproteins has been demonstrated in the target cells and in cell-free systems. Certain polyribonucleotides can bind S-R and promote the release of S-R complexes from DNA; this effect is dependent on the nucleotide sequence of the RNA.

A test of a hypothetical model for RNA-binding and intracellular dynamics of steroid-receptor complexes. In our working model, an A-R complex binds to the transcriptional complex on a responsive gene and promotes RNA synthesis. By binding to the RNA product, the A-R complex and RNA may be released from the target gene, allowing the gene to participate in further RNA synthesis. RNA bound to the A-R complex may be processed/stabilized and transported out of nucleus for participation in protein synthesis. Removal of RNA from the receptor complex is required for the A-R complex to recycle back to chromatin. Our experiments showed that if RNA synthesis was inhibited by actinomycin D, the A-R complex accumulated as a chromatin-bound form. In the presence of 3′-deoxyadenosine (3′dA), a potent inhibitor of RNA polyadenylation and nucleo-cytoplasmic RNA transport, the A-R complex was maintained in a non-DNA-binding form in the cytosol fraction, and recycling of the A-R complex appeared to be prevented. The level of chromatin-bound A-R complexes was reduced.

It is not possible to eliminate the possibility that 3′-dA exerts its effect on the transformation and recycling of A-R complexes through mechanisms that are not directly related to RNA synthesis or processing. 3′-dA has been shown to affect nuclear RNA methylation and chromosomal protein phosphorylation. Phosphorylation of AR and other SRs and associated proteins has been studied, although the precise role of protein phosphorylation and other structural changes during receptor transformation remains uncertain.

Immunochemical Studies of Androgen Receptors

Poly- and monoclonal anti-AR antibodies. We have found that circulating autoantibodies to ARs and 5α-reductase are present at high titers in the blood sera of some prostate cancer patients. Autoanti-AR antibodies from prostate cancer patients were AR-specific and did not interact with GR, PR, or ER. Because of their specificity, these autoantibodies were used to verify that the proteins made in cell-free systems from AR cDNA were ARs. After we obtained AR-cDNAs, we employed a molecular fusion technique to obtain large quantities of specific AR polypeptides linked to a *E. coli* protein, *trpE.* Polyclonal anti-AR antibodies were obtained from rabbits immunized with fusion proteins that represent different domains of AR. Spleen cells from immunized rats were fused with SP2/0 myeloma cells to produce hybridomas secreting monoclonal anti-AR antibodies specific for AR. One of the monoclonal antibodies we produced recognized an epitope in the amino terminal domain adjacent to the DNA-binding domain.

Immunocytolocalization of AR. Polyclonal and monoclonal antibodies against AR have been used for the immunocytolocalization of ARs in target cells. In rat and human prostates as well as in monkey seminal vesicles, most of the AR was found in epithelial cell nuclei. In monkey seminal vesicles, both AR and ER were found in the same stromal cell nuclei (ER was not seen in epithelial cell nuclei), indicating that both ER and AR may be involved in the control of stromal cell function. In foreskin and other skin cells, AR was also found to localize in nuclei. In rat brain, the highest number of AR-immunoreactive neurons were found in the hypothalamus and cortical and limbic system structures. We have also found that AR was present in both the nuclear and cytoplasmic compartment of motor neurons. Using Northern analysis and immunoblotting, we also studied AR expression by rat sebaceous glands. Electron microscopic immunogold labeling showed AR to be concentrated largely in the perinuclear regions of basal cells of the preputial gland to the same or greater extent than in the prostate.

Positive and Negative Regulation of Gene Expression

To regulate the growth of target organs, androgens can stimulate the expression of certain genes but also repress the expression of other genes simultaneously. Genes for proteins listed below have been useful in the study of the growth and function of rat ventral prostate. The positive and negative regulation of the levels of mRNAs for 3 of these protein markers in the ventral prostate of rats after castration and injection of DHT is shown in figure 1-5.

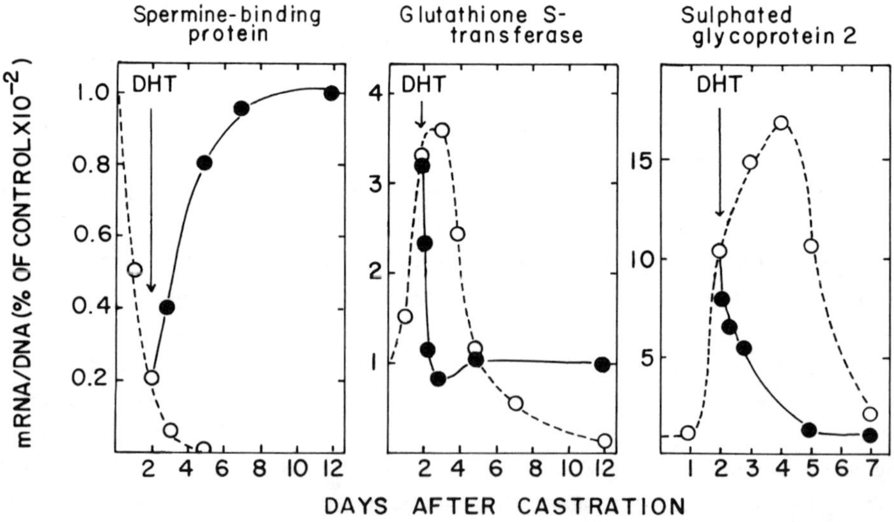

Figure 1-5. Levels of mRNAs of spermine-binding protein, glutathione S-transferase, and sulphated glycoprotein 2 in rat ventral prostate after castration and injection of DHT.

Positive Regulation

α-Protein. This androgen-dependent protein of rat ventral prostate was originally discovered in our laboratory in 1971. Other investigators have also rediscovered the same protein, naming it as *prostate-binding protein, prostatein,* and *estramustine-binding protein.* The protein is the major secretory protein (>40%) in the prostate fluid. The protein, which is cholesterol-binding, has 4 polypeptide subunits. cDNA has been constructed and androgen dependency for the synthesis of its mRNA has been studied extensively by many investigators. A small quantity of a similar protein may be present in human prostate.

Prostatic spermine-binding protein (SBP). We have cloned and sequenced the cDNA for this protein, which we found in 1977 as a specific polyamine-binding protein whose synthesis is stimulated by androgen. To confirm the amino acid sequence deduced from cDNA, we also sequenced the purified protein. Because the amino terminus of the protein was blocked, we employed fast atom bombardment mass spectrometry, tandem mass spectometry, and conventional sequencing methods to establish the amino-terminal sequence of the protein. From protein sequencing, we identified a section of cDNA that was "missing" in the initial cDNA coding for SBP. A similar protein is present in mouse prostate.

For Negative Regulation

Glutathione S-transferase (GST). Androgens, while stimulating the production of certain proteins, can also repress the levels of a limited number of mRNAs that code for at least 4 proteins with molecular weights of 29, 37, 46, and 49 kDa. By cDNA cloning and sequencing, we found that the 29 kDa protein is the Yb_1 subunit of GST. Yb forms of GST have been colocalized with uridylic acid-rich small nuclear RNAs at interchromatinic regions of the cell nucleus.

Sulphated glycoprotein 2 (SGP-2). By cloning and sequencing cDNA, we have identified the 49 kDa androgen-repressed protein as SGP-2. Northern-blot analysis of ventral prostate indicated that the mRNA increased 17-fold 4 days after castration. A rapid decrease in the concentration of this mRNA was observed within 6 hr after a single injection of DHT into castrated rats. Of the 16 male and female organs analyzed, only the ventral prostate showed such a large effect.

Conclusion

Prostate functions have often been evaluated by measurement of the levels of marker proteins and their mRNAs. For example, Chung Lee and associates have shown that, in normal rats, cell proliferation occurred in distal segments, whereas sulphated glycoprotein 2 and cathepsin D (2 marker proteins for cells undergoing programmed death) were actively produced by cells at the proximal region of the prostate duct system. After castration, the level of these 2 proteins decreased at the proximal region and increased at the distal region, indicating that the cell degeneration pattern shifted from the proximal region to the distal region. This interesting phenomenon may be related to mechanisms involving prostate cell homeostasis.

Neuroendocrine systems may have a regulatory role in normal and diseased prostate function. Leland Chung et al have used rat ventral prostate fragments implanted under the renal capsules of syngeneic rats to study the production of secretory protein in the denervated prostate. The denervated prostate had a reduced level of α-protein production, but this decrease was restored by the administration of exogenous androgen and/or a β-adrenergic agonist, isoproterenol. The observation suggested that androgens can also act through β-adrenergic receptor pathways.

Bibliography

1. Liao S, Kokontis J, Sai T, Hiipakka RA. Androgen receptors: structures, mutations, antibodies and cellular dynamics. J Steroid Biochem 1989; 34:41-51.
2. Bettuzzi S, Hiipakka RA, Gilna P, Liao S. Identification of the androgen-repressed mRNA for a 48-kilodalton prostate protein as sulfated glycoprotein 2 by cDNA cloning and sequence analysis. Biochem J 1989; 257:293-96.
3. Chang C, Whelan CT, Popovich TC, Kokontis J, Liao S. Fusion proteins containing androgen receptor sequences and their use in the production of poly- and monoclonal anti-androgen receptor antibodies. Endocrinology 1989; 123:1097-99.
4. Imperato-McGinley J, Ip NY, Gautier T, et al. DNA linkage analysis and studies of the androgen receptor gene in a large kindred with complete androgen insensitivity. Am J Med Genet 1990; 36:104-08.
5. Sai T, Seino S, Chang C, et al. An exonic point mutation of the androgen receptor gene in a family with complete androgen insensitivity. Am J Human Genetics 1990; 46:1095-1100.
6. West NB, Chang C, Liao S, Brenner RM. Localization and regulation of estrogen, progestin, and androgen receptors in the seminal vesicle of the Rhesus monkey. J Steroid Biochem Mol Biol 1990; 37:11-21.
7. Liang T, Hiipakka RA, Stebbins J, Liao S. Anti-5α-reductase autoantibodies in the serum of patients with prostatic cancer. J Clin Endocrinol Metabol 1990; 71:1666-72.
8. Lee C, Sensibar JA, Dudek SM, Hiipakka RA, Liao S. Prostatic ductal system in rats: Regional variation in morphological and functional activities. Biol Reprod 1990; 43:1079-86.
9. Guthrie PD, Freeman MR, Liao S, Chung LWK. Regulation of gene expression in rat prostate by androgen and β-adrenergic receptor pathways. Mol Endocrinol 1990; 4:1343-53.
10. He WW, Fischer LM, Sun S, et al. Molecular cloning of androgen receptors from divergent species with a polymerase chain reaction technique: complete cDNA sequence of the mouse androgen receptor and isolation of androgen receptor cDNA probes from frog, guinea pig, and clawed frog. Biochem Biophys Res Commun 1990; 171:697-704.
11. Kokontis J, Ito K, Hiipakka RA, Liao S. Expression and function of normal and LNCaP androgen receptors in androgen-insensitive human prostatic cancer cells: altered hormone and antihormone specificity in gene transactivation. Receptor (in press).

2

GROWTH REQUIREMENTS OF HUMAN PROSTATE CANCERS IN VITRO AND IN VIVO

James M. Kozlowski, M.D., F.A.C.S.; Debra M. Sutkowski; Xianglin Liu, M.D.; Chau-Jye Fong, M.D.; Edward R. Sherwood, Ph.D.; and Chung Lee, Ph.D.

Introduction

ADENOCARCINOMA OF THE PROSTATE is the most common cancer among American men, with recent estimates suggesting that it will account for 22% (122,000 cases) of newly diagnosed cancer in 1991.[1] Advanced stage disease (C, D1, D2) will be identified in more than 40% of these cases.[2] Annual progression rates of 10-12% can be anticipated for patients with untreated stage C disease, of whom about 60% will exhibit evidence of disease progression at 5 yr.[3] Similarily, about 85% of patients with stage D1 disease exhibit progression within 5 yr, whereas those with stage D2 disease have a median survival of about 30 mo, with an anticipated 5-yr survival approaching 20%.[4] The biological ramifications of these statistics are best appreciated when one considers that prostate cancer will account for 12% (32,000 cases) of male cancer deaths in 1991 and is now the second leading cause of cancer mortality in that population.[1]

These epidemiologic observations serve to emphasize that adenocarcinoma of the prostate is a major factor in the health of the male population of the United States. Tumors contained within the confines of the anatomic capsule (stages A, B) may

These studies were supported in part by NIH grant DK39250, contract CM97628, from the National Cancer Institute, and by the Lucy and Edwin Kretschmer Fund of Northwestern University Medical School.

The authors wish to thank Carole Herhold for her invaluable assistance in the preparation of this manuscript and Dr. John T. Grayhack for his leadership, support, and insight.

be curable with either radical prostatectomy or radiation therapy. Unfortunately, the prospects are not as favorable for patients with advanced stage tumors. Admittedly, about 70% of such patients will exhibit beneficial responses of an objective and subjective nature to androgen deprivation. The efficacy of androgen ablation, documented in the landmark observations of Huggins and Hodges in 1941, was based upon their hypothesis that prostate cancer cells retained certain characteristics of nontransformed prostatic epithelium and would likely undergo atrophy following androgen deprivation.[5] Unfortunately, the duration of this response ranges from several months to several years, with the majority of such patients succumbing to the uncontrolled proliferation of androgen-independent tumor populations (stage D3) within 6-18 mo.[4]

To date, there is no effective systemic therapy for the treatment of advanced stage, androgen-refractory prostate cancer. Numerous attempts have been made to treat these tumors with single-agent and multiagent chemotherapy. Unfortunately, only 10% of such patients exhibit evidence of partial, objective disease regression, and the majority of such patients demonstrate evidence of disease progression within 3-6 mo.[2,4]

An urgent scientific and clinical need exists for the identification of new and effective treatment strategies for the management of disseminated prostate cancer. Unfortunately, our basic perceptions concerning the biology of prostate cancer remain quite primitive. In large part, this lack of insight may be attributed to the complexity inherent in the biology of normal, hyperplastic, and malignant human prostate systems. This acknowledged deficit is further compounded by the lack of suitable in vitro and in vivo (animal) models that would permit a detailed, repetitive, and multiphenotypic investigation of the critical biological questions that remain to be answered. This paper will focus on the issues of heterogeneity within human prostate systems and summarize some of the methodological approaches used by our laboratory to further dissect the biology of these most intriguing neoplasms.

The Zonal, Cellular, and Phenotypic Heterogeneity of the Prostate and Prostate Cancers

The elegant anatomic studies conducted by McNeal have demonstrated that the human prostate gland can be separated into 4 distinct regions or zones. The peripheral zone constitutes about 75% of the glandular prostate, with its ductal system entering along the posterolateral recesses of the distal urethra from the prostatic apex to the verumonantum. Most prostate cancers appear to originate within this region. The central zone occupies 20% of the glandular prostate, and its ductal network follows the route of the ejaculatory ducts to the urethra. The transition zone accounts for 4-5% of the glandular prostate. It consists of 2 small lobules of tissue lateral to the preprostatic sphincter. Benign prostatic hyperplasia (BPH) originates from this area.[6] Stage A1 prostate cancers may also emanate from this zone.[7] The final anatomically discrete zone within the glandular prostate is the periurethral gland region, which represents 1% of the total volume of the glandular prostate. It is of interest that these various regions appear to have differing acinar, stromal, and cellular configurations. The anatomical and histological similarities shared by the peripheral zone, transition zone, and periuretheral gland region may be attributable to a common embryonic origin from the urogenital sinus. Similarly, close association between the central glandular zone, the ejaculatory ducts, and the seminal vesicles may reflect a common origin from the mesonephric duct. Finally, this consideration of the zonal heterogeneity of the human prostate would be deficient without mention of the ventral fibromuscular stroma, which represents over 30% of the tissue within the prostatic capsule. It is composed predominantly of smooth muscle fibers that maintain continuity proximally with the detrusor muscle of the bladder neck.[8] It is readily apparent that an elucidation of the biological features unique to the peripheral and transition zone regions would provide seminal insight into the pathogenesis of prostate cancer and BPH, respectively.

Normal and pathologic human prostate glands also exhibit heterogeneity with respect to their epithelial and stromal composition. The epithelial compartment consists of adluminal (secretory), basal, ductal epithelial, and endocrine-paracrine cellular subsets.[6] Numerous morphological and biochemical features serve to distinguish the various members of the epithelial compartment.[9] For example, the secretory cells react with monoclonal antibodies to prostate-specific antigen (PSA) and prostatic acid phosphatase (PAP). Basal cells are not highlighted with these monoclonal antibodies. It is theorized that the basal cell compartment functions primarily as reserve cells and is responsible for tissue repair observed following infarction and infection.

It has also been speculated that the epithelial hyperplasia noted in BPH is due to the proliferative activity of basal cells, but these perceptions remain hypothetical. It has been suggested that the endocrine-paracrine cells may play a role in both BPH and prostate cancer.[10] Although most of these cells contain serotonin and probe positively for neuron-specific enolase, silver stains and other immunocytohistochemical techniques have also defined the presence of cells positive for argyrophil, argentaffin, and somatostatin.

The stromal compartment also consists of a diverse array of cellular subsets including fibroblasts, smooth muscle cells, and skeletal muscle elements. In fact, the capsular septa and stroma comprise a dynamic scaffolding system for the underlying prostatic parenchyma and, as a composite unit, constitute between 25-30% of the total volume of the prostate gland.[9] The fibroblasts tend to be organized parallel to the long axis of the tubulosaccular glands and tend to form a more predictable relationship to the basement membrane. The abundant smooth muscle surrounding individual glands is thought to play an important role in the release of glandular secretions and contributes to the functional integrity of the internal urethral sphincter. In addition to these well-recognized structural and functional roles, the prostatic stroma is thought to play a dynamic role in the pathogenesis of BPH via the elaboration of mitogenic signals that induce proliferative activity within the epithelial compartment.[6,8,9] Similar aberrations in stromal-epithelial interaction have been postulated to play a role in the evolution of prostate cancer.[11]

In addition to this zonal and cellular heterogeneity, numerous examples exist that typify the intercellular heterogeneity in the normal, hyperplastic, and malignant human prostate. For example, recent studies have demonstrated that the adluminal and basal cells are distinguished on the basis of their expression of specific cytokeratins.[12,13] The latter are a class of cytoskeletal intermediate filaments found in epithelial and mesothelial cells. Each type of epithelial cell possesses a distinct profile of cytokeratin (CK) polypeptides. For example, CK polypeptides 5, 7, 8, 15, 18, and 19 can be demonstrated in normal and hyperplastic human prostate glands. In distinction, established prostate cancer cell lines (PC-3, DU-145, and LNCaP) and fresh prostate cancers show expression of CKs 8 and 18 but not CKs 5, 7, and 15, which are observed only in the benign prostate.[12,13] Interestingly, no apparent qualitative differences have been detected with respect to CK expression when a comparison is made between central and peripheral zone tissues.[13] Furthermore, numerous studies have demonstrated that CK5 is selectively expressed in the basal cell population of the human prostate.[13,14] CK5 is not expressed in prostate cancer specimens, leading to the speculation that carcinomas arise from a malignant transformation within the adluminal epithelial cell compartment. These perceptions are further validated by immunohistochemical studies using the monoclonal anticytokeratin 8.12, which exhibits immunoreactivity with the basal—but not the secretory—epithelial cells of the fetal, juvenile, normal adult, and hyperplastic prostate. The 8.12 antibody does not stain prostate cancer tissues, further supporting the hypothesis that prostate cancers arise within the secretory cell compartment.[13,14]

Perhaps the most pivotal question regarding phenotypic heterogeneity concerns the emergence of androgen-dependent, androgen-sensitive, and androgen-independent tumor subpopulations. It has been speculated that the emergence of such heterogeneity may involve 1 of 2 potential mechanisms. In the adaptation model, prostate tumors are viewed as initially homogenous with respect to androgen sensitivity. Hormonal ablation would then induce changes in the host environment, leading to the development of androgen-resistant clones via the mechanism of adaptive transformation.

Conversely, the clonal selection model assumes that prostate cancers become heterogeneous immediately following malignant transformation because of genomic perturbations that arise due to the genetic instability intrinsic to most tumor systems.[4] By using the transplantable Dunning R3327 H rat prostatic carcinoma model, Isaacs and Coffey demonstrated that the mechanism responsible for the emergence of androgen resistance is indeed the intrinsic heterogeneity of the original prostate cancer, thus validating the clonal selection theory.[15]

In prostate cancer systems, a wide variety of phenotypes have been identified that may distinguish biologically indolent tumors from those possessing invasive or metastatic properties, including:

- High tumor grade
- Increasing Gleason score
- Tumor volume >1 cc
- The presence of aneuploidy

- Pretreatment serum testosterone values of <300 mg/dl
- >6 areas of increased uptake on a bone scan
- Nuclear androgen receptor levels <110 fmol/mg of DNA
- Abnormal nuclear roundness factor
- Aberrations of nucleolar size and pleomorphism
- Amplified oncogene expression
- Exaggerated production of urokinase-type plasminogen activator
- Increased tumor cell motility
- Negative cell-surface charge.[4]

The Tissue Matrix System: The Role of Stromal-Epithelial Interaction

An impressive amount of evidence has accumulated suggesting that mesenchymal-epithelial interactions play a strategic role in the androgen-induced morphogenesis and growth of embryonic and adult prostatic tissue.[16,17] The mature secretory epithelium of the human prostate consists of highly differentiated cells residing in a complex environment in which factors such as circulating androgens, extracellular matrix, stroma, and growth factors may dynamically influence the phenotypes of cellular growth and differentiation.

Epithelial cells attach preferentially to basement membrane extracellular matrix. The latter is composed of the unique collagen substrate (type 4), the attachment of glycoprotein laminin (with lesser amounts of enactin and nidogen), and heparan sulfate proteoglycan.[18] These extracellular matrix (ECM) components play a fundamental role in the anchorage of epithelial cells to the underlying substratum and determine their ultimate shape and polarity. The ECM may dynamically affect the ability of epithelial cells to respond to various growth factors. Indeed, maintenance of normal cell polarity is necessary for the optimal expression of growth factor receptors, which reside preferentially along the posterolateral cell surface.[19] Additional evidence suggests that ECM components play an active role in the control of gene expression and may have a profound impact upon cellular morphology and function by inducing a redistribution of the cytoskeleton.[20] Some ECM preparations may sequester heparin-binding growth factors (such as basic fibroblast growth factor) due to the affinity of these growth factors for the proteoglycan component of basement membrane.[21,22] Finally, it has been proposed that such tissue-matrix interactions may have an equally important role with respect to prostate carcinogenesis.[23,24]

Inadequacy of Existing In Vitro and In Vivo Models of Human Prostate Cancer

The preceding discussion summarized some of the salient features typifying the zonal, cellular, and phenotypic heterogeneity relevant to benign and malignant prostate systems. The complexity of such interactional dynamics and our inadequate understanding of the critical biological events involved are the factors primarily responsible for the scarcity of useful in vitro and in vivo models of human prostate cancer. It should be emphasized that important information has been forthcoming from investigations performed using rodent models of human prostate cancer, which include the Noble,[25] ACI,[26] Pollard,[27] and Dunning R3327 tumors.[15] Despite their utility, observations performed on such systems cannot substitute for a multiphenotypic analysis of human prostate cancer.[28]

Attempts to cultivate and serially passage human prostate cancer cells in tissue culture have met with numerous methodological frustrations. These difficulties readily explain the scarcity of well-characterized, immortalized cell lines derived from patients with prostate cancer such as PC-3,[29] DU-145,[30] LNCaP,[31] and PPC-1.[32]

It should be emphasized that cell lines PC-3, DU-145, and PPC-1 are completely androgen-independent. They are capable of sustained proliferation in the absence of exogenous dihydrotestosterone (DHT). Moreover, they neither express nor secrete the biochemical markers prototypic of prostatic epitheliality, namely PAP and PSA. LNCaP is androgen-sensitive in that its proliferative activity is amplified in the presence of exogenous DHT.[33,34] However, it is capable of basal growth in the absence of androgen. Perhaps in concert with its demonstrated androgen sensitivity, LNCaP has maintained its ability to express—albeit in heterogeneous fashion—both PAP and PSA.[35]

A brief analysis of the biographical history underlying the establishment of these cell lines sheds important light on the behavioral nuances exhibited by these tumor systems. PC-3, DU-145, and LNCaP were derived from metastatic foci, namely bone marrow, brain, and supraclavicular lymph node, respectively. Moreover, all of the patients from whom these tumors were extracted had undergone androgen-ablative therapy. Thus, from their conception, these tumor cell lines were preselected for their absolute or relative androgen insensitivity. PPC-1 was derived following a "channel" transurethral resection of the prostate in a patient with a high Gleason histotype tumor associated with obstruction of the bladder neck and widespread metastasis. Despite their origins from aggressive tumor systems, only PC-3 and PPC-1 appear to be highly tumorigenic in the nude mouse model.[32,36] PC-3 has been rigorously assessed and shown to maintain a highly invasive/metastatic phenotype in vivo.[28,36-38]

Not surprisingly, the heterotransplantation of fresh human prostatic tumors into immune-deficient animals has also proven to be exceedingly difficult. It has been estimated that only 1% of such fresh tumor specimens exhibit a limited capacity for xenografting. Consequently, there is a scarcity of well-characterized in vivo transplantable human prostatic tumor lines. Those in existence include the androgen-dependent tumor systems designated PC-82[39] and HONDA.[40] These systems are completely androgen-dependent and will not grow in female nude mice or in castrated males. Again, an analysis of the clinical biography underlying the establishment of these systems sheds important light on their biological behavior. For example, PC-82 was derived from a primary tumor following radical perineal prostatectomy and had not undergone clinical "preselection," a factor that may explain maintenance of androgen dependency. HONDA was derived from a prostate cancer metastatic to the testis. Obviously, the latter organ provided an androgen-enriched environment, which might explain the unique androgen dependency of this tumor.

Propagation and Phenotypic Dissection of Human Prostate Cancers In Vitro

Our laboratory is actively pursuing a variety of approaches designed to enhance in vitro cultivation of fresh human prostate cancers. Prior to embarking on this admittedly difficult task, we performed a thorough evaluation of several established human prostate cancer cell lines in the hope that insights derived from such an analysis would assist in the optimization of the in vitro growth milieu for fresh prostate cancer systems. Only a small sampling of the many characterization studies will be highlighted in the following paragraphs.

PC-3 is an androgen-independent prostatic carcinoma cell line that has been the focus of numerous investigative efforts by our laboratory.[28,36-38,41] It is known to exhibit autonomous growth in vitro and possesses both the invasive and metastatic phenotype when assessed in the Boyden chamber chemoinvasion assay and nude mouse model, respectively.[28,36,42] We have recently documented that PC-3 cells synthesize and secrete growth factors into their conditioned medium that are highly mitogenic for the more biologically indolent cell lines DU-145 and LNCaP.[41] Following this observation, the conditioned medium was dialyzed against distilled water (4°C) using a 3.5 kD cutoff membrane and lyophilized. Gel filtration chromatography then performed on this conditioned medium preparation revealed the major peak of mitogenic activity at 5-10 kD. Synthesis/secretion of TGF-α was confirmed by immunoblotting and radioimmunoassay.

EGF receptors (K_d = 5.3 n*M*) were detected on PC-3 cells by radio receptor analysis. The addition of neutralizing antibodies to TGF-α effectively abrogated the mitogenic impact of the 5-10 kD fraction of PC-3 conditioned medium. Moreover, antibodies to TGF-α and/or the EGF receptor inhibited the proliferation of PC-3 cells under serum-free defined conditions (figure 2-1). As a composite, these observations fulfill the necessary requirements for the existence of an external autocrine growth factor mechanism, since documentation of the latter requires (1) the synthesis and secretion of an endogenous growth factor, (2) the presence of cell-surface receptors for the growth factor, and (3) the induction of cellular proliferation following ligand-receptor binding.

It should be emphasized, however, that PC-3 growth was incompletely abrogated by the addition of anti-TGF-α and/or anti-EGF receptor antibodies. This suggests that other mechanisms of autonomous growth regulation play an active role in maintaining the proliferative drive of the PC-3 cell line. Finally, these studies suggest that

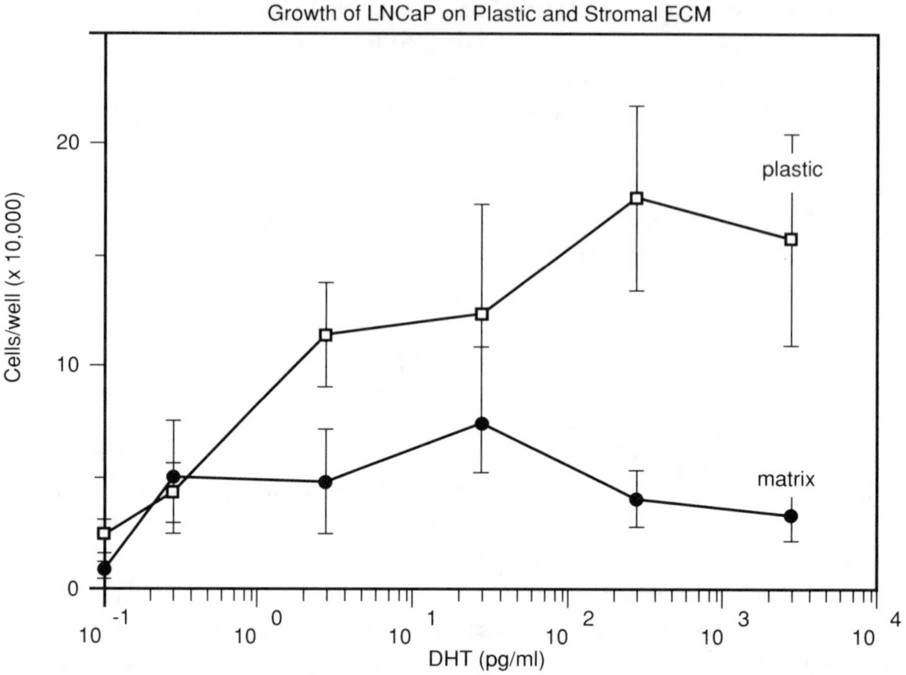

Figure 2-1. Analysis of LNCaP cell growth in response to increasing concentrations of DHT. LNCaP cells were cultured on tissue culture plastic or stromal ECM in the presence of DHT ranging in concentration from 0-2000 pg/ml. On day 6, cells were detached from the culture surface and counted using a hemacytometer to determine cellular proliferation. N = 8-12/group.

the addition of exogenous TGF-α or mitogen-enriched fractions of PC-3 conditioned medium might be advantageous for the growth and propagation of fresh prostate tumor systems in vitro.

In contrast, experimental studies involving the androgen-sensitive prostate cancer cell line LNCaP were designed to probe the impact of various in vitro conditions on the phenotypes of proliferation and differentiation. LNCaP is ideally suited for this purpose because it is capable of slow, sustained growth in the absence of androgen but responds to the administration of exogenous DHT to increase proliferative activity. Moreover, it has retained the ability to synthesize and secrete PAP and PSA, making it an exquisitely useful target to evaluate those in vitro conditions favoring the differentiated phenotype.

Along these lines, earlier studies performed in our laboratory demonstrated that BPH epithelial cells grown in monolayer tissue culture on a plastic substrate undergo rapid proliferation and lose their ability to synthesize and secrete PAP and PSA. However, when these epithelial cells are grown on a basement membrane extracellular matrix (Matrigel), cell growth is markedly curtailed but the secretion of PAP/PSA is significantly increased. Morphological studies demonstrated that cells grown on plastic formed monolayer cultures, whereas those cultivated on extracellular matrix developed very distinct organoid-like clusters, further suggesting the induction of a differentiated pheonotype.[43]

Similar observations have been forthcoming in our studies of the LNCaP tumor system.[35] In this case, tumor cells were grown either on a plastic substrate or extracellular matrix generated from BPH stromal cells. The addition of increasing concentrations of DHT stimulated the growth of LNCaP cells cultivated under both experimental conditions (figure 2-1). However, those cells on tissue culture plastic exhibited far greater proliferative activity. Conversely, there was a striking dichotomy with respect to androgen-induced secretion of PAP and PSA (figure 2-2). LNCaP cells cultivated on stromal matrix synthesized and secreted far greater quantities of PAP and PSA when compared to those cultivated on tissue culture plastic. These experiments suggest that androgen-sensitive prostate cancer systems retain certain features considered prototypic of nontransformed prostatic epithelial cells. Furthermore, these studies suggest that the use of natural substrates may be advantageous for promotion of androgen-regulated growth/differentiation of androgen-sensitive prostate tumor systems.

The limited scope of this paper precludes a detailed delineation of numerous experimental strategies being employed by our laboratory to promote the growth and propagation of human prostate cancers in vitro. The remainder of this section will briefly summarize some of the more important methodological issues, such as (1) tissue acquisition, (2) tissue processing, (3) media composition, (4) choice of growth substrate, (5) methods of expansion, and (6) characterization strategies.

It seems intuitively clear that the prompt acquisition and expeditious processing of fresh prostate cancer tissue is highly desirable. There are a number of potential sources of human prostate cancer, including:

- Needle aspiration/biopsy of the tumor primary in vivo
- Radical prostatectomy specimens
- "Channel" transurethral resection of the prostate
- Materials derived following pelvic lymph node dissection
- Biopsy of subcutaneous lymph nodes/visceral metasteses
- Bone marrow aspiration/biopsy
- Fresh autopsy.

Background analysis of existing prostate cancer cell lines suggests that the most desirable tumor target is one that is derived from high Gleason histotype tumors that have already exhibited a propensity for local invasion and/or systemic dissemination. In addition, it is desirable to process sizable amounts of tissue (2-3 g) that can be harvested under aseptic conditions. The latter contingency frequently precludes the utility of aspiration/biopsy specimens obtained via transrectal biopsy.

In most instances, modest amounts of solid tumor material will be available for scientific purposes. Even materials derived from metastatic foci will be heterogeneous and contain admixtures of epithelial and stromal elements. Further processing

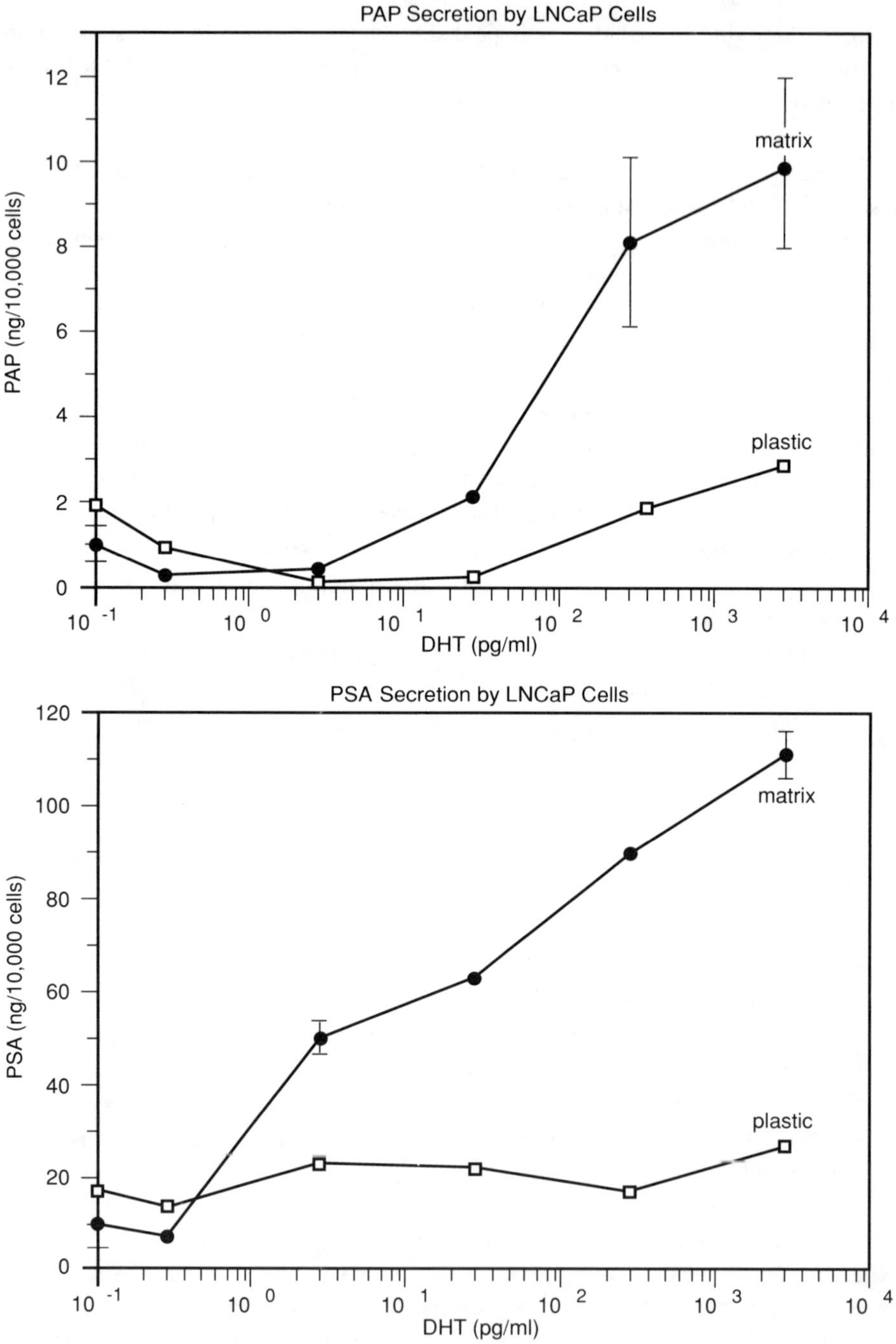

Figure 2-2. Analysis of LNCaP cell secretion of PAP/PSA in response to increasing concentration of DHT. LNCaP cells were cultured on tissue culture plastic or stromal ECM in the presence of DHT ranging in concentration from 0-2000 pg/ml. On day 6, conditioned media were harvested for PAP/PSA analysis using an immunoradiometric assay.

will require (1) meticulous mechanical disaggregation; (2) the culture of "spill-over" cells, which frequently represents an "epithelial-rich" suspension; (3) the initiation of fragment culture on plastic/natural substrates; and (4) a 4-hr enzymatic dissociation of the remaining tissue fragments and the use of type I collagenase (200 U/ml) and DNAse (100 μg/ml). Bone marrow aspirates performed near sites of skeletal metastases (as defined by bone scan imaging) have been reported to yield a mean of 4.5 x 10^7 viable nucleated cells, 52% of which demonstrate growth in semisolid agar.[44] Furthermore, a panel of immunocytochemical probes can be used to validate the presence of prostate cancer cells.[45] Obviously, such aspirates can be further enriched with cell separation techniques and rapidly incorporated into in vitro culture.

In most cases, we have made deliberate attempts to establish fragment and monolayer culture systems (figures 2-3A and 2-3B). Because most of the established prostate cancer cell lines were derived from fragment culture systems, the potential importance of this rather simple technique should not be overlooked.[46] Depending on tissue availability, we have made aggressive attempts to establish fragment cultures on tissue culture plastic, floating collagen gels, and other natural (biological) substrates. With respect to the latter, we employ collagen type I/II, laminin, fibronectin, basement membrane extracellular matrix (Matrigel), and extracellular matrix derived from BPH/cancer stroma.[28,47]

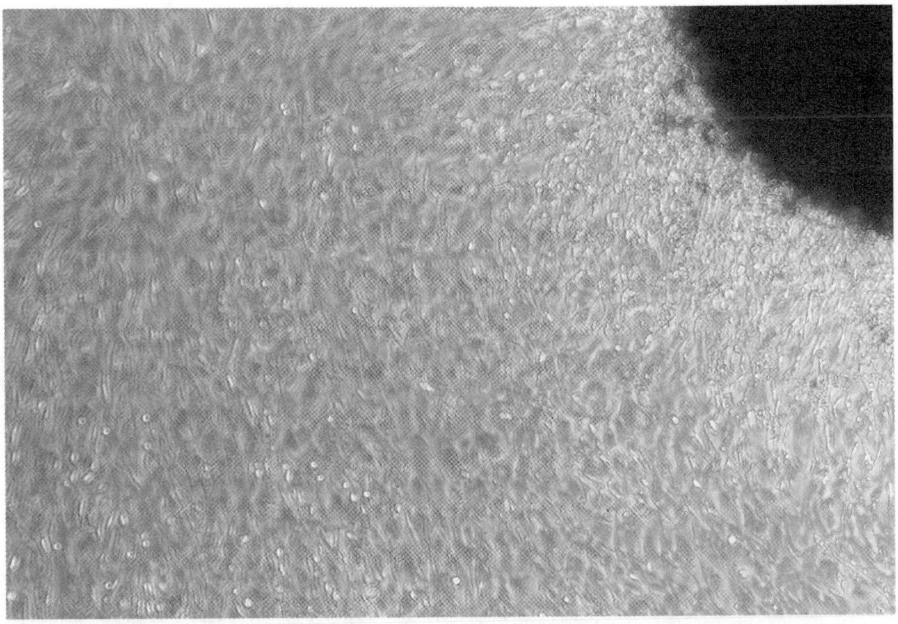

Figure 2-3A. Phase contrast micrograph of a fresh prostate cancer fragment culture on specialized collagen gel. Tissue fragments (3–5 1 mm^3) were plated onto the collagen surface, where they adhere or embed in the loose fiber structure of the gel. Serum-free media supplemented with growth factors is added until the upper portion of the tissue is reached but not covered.

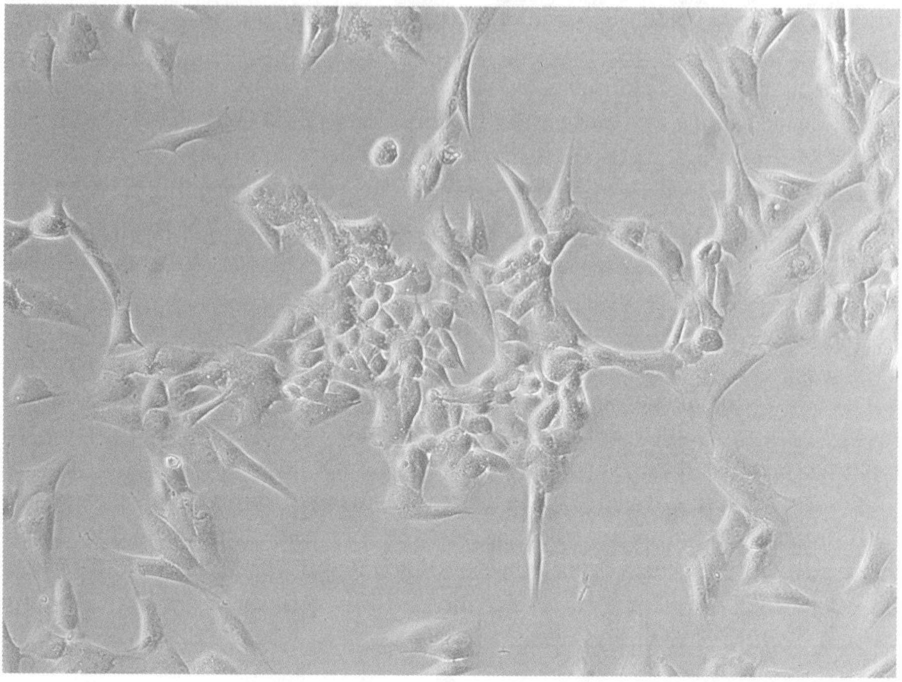

Figure 2-3B. Phase contrast micrograph of fresh prostate cancer epithelial cells cultured on plastic. Tissue fragments were minced into 1 mm^3 fragments and dissociated with 200 U/ml collagenase type I and 100 μg/ml DNAse type I in RPMI-1640 media with 10% fetal bovine serum. Following gentle agitation for 4 hr at 37°C, the resulting cell suspension was washed with phosphate-buffered saline and plated in 25 cm^2 tissue culture flasks.

Naturally, cell suspensions generated following enzymatic dissociation are processed in a somewhat different manner. Ideally, the effective separation of epithelial and stromal components would facilitate the selective propagation, expansion, and analysis of these cellular subsets. Moreover, the isolation of acinar and stromal elements with a high degree of purity would greatly enhance investigation of mechanisms underlying glandular stromal interaction. Our laboratory has developed a modification of a 5-step discontinuous Percoll gradient technique that permits the separation of stromal/epithelial elements with a high degree of purity.[12,28]

Unfortunately, the small amount of tumor tissue available for experimental purposes frequently precludes such gradient-separation techniques. Therefore, heterogeneous cell suspensions are plated as monolayers on plastic substrates (25 cm^3 flasks) and on the above-mentioned spectrum of natural substrates. It is our current perception that prostate cancer epithelial cells must be separated from the stromal "passengers" as soon as possible. In order to accomplish this goal, we have employed the technique of "differential" trypsinization. The latter permits the relatively selective detachment of stromal cells, which can be subcultured.

Our laboratory and others have reported on the utility of serum-free medium preparations for the propagation of prostatic epithelial cells in finite tissue culture.[12,28,48,49] The use of serum-free medium (SFM) is desirable for a number of reasons, including the following:

1. It avoids the lot-to-lot variability associated with the use of serum.
2. Serum can be toxic in high concentrations.
3. Serum may distort specialized cellular functions.
4. The use of SFM decreases the risk of contamination.
5. Serum may exert undesirable "selection pressure" on cells.[50]

Several SFM formulations have been defined specifically for the cultivation of human prostatic epithelial cells that include WAJC-404 and PFMR-4.[48,50,51] Each has evolved along slightly different lines as modifications of Ham's F-12 medium. An important constituent of these basic nutrient formulations is a relatively low ionic calcium concentration ($\leq$ 0.13 m*M*). Under serum-free conditions, the latter has been shown to be essential for the establishment of single-cell suspensions, for normal cell attachment to the plastic substratum, and for the detachment of the cellular monolayer into single cells following treatment with collagenase.[48]

Studies emanating from our laboratory regarding the phenotypic characterization of BPH epithelial cells involved a modification of the WAJC-404 medium plus essential growth factors/additives popularized by McKeehan.[48,49] The specific additives are detailed in table 2-1. Bovine pituitary extract (BPE) appears to be a strategic supplemental ingredient and probably provides an enriched source of acidic fibroblast growth factor (FGF-α).[52-54] Cholera toxin, which appears to be a potent mitogen for prostate epithelial cells cultivated in SFM, acts by increasing intracellular CAMP levels. Polyvinylpyrrolidone (PVP) is a form of synthetic albumin used in place of human serum albumin in some of our media formulations. Although DHT appears

Table 2-1. Additives to the Serum-Free Media Used to Propagate Prostate Epithelial Cells

"Complete" WAJC-404 Medium	
Insulin	5 μg/ml
Transferrin	5 μg/ml
Selenous acid	5 ng/ml
Bovine pituitary extract	30 μg/ml
Prolactin	2.3 μg/ml
Epidermal growth factor	10 ng/ml
Cholera toxin	10 ng/ml
Dexamethasone	1×10^{-10} M
Dihydrotestosterone	1×10^{-10} M
Polyvinyl pyrrolidone	2 mg/ml
Penicillin	100 U/ml
Streptomycin	100 μg/ml

to play a strategic role in the maintenance, differentiation, and proliferation of human prostate tissues in vivo, most reports have failed to establish its role as an essential mitogen for prostate epithelial cells in vitro. However, because it increases the proliferation of LNCaP in vitro, we have chosen to maintain androgen in our medium formulation. Of interest, when stromal/epithelial relationships are maintained (i.e., organ culture), exogenous DHT has been shown to exert its anticipated influence on the phenotypes of proliferation/differentiation.[35,43]

To date, it has not been possible to sustain the growth of fresh human prostate cancer systems in vitro using growth-factor enriched serum-free medium. At present, the addition of fetal bovine serum (10-20%) is necessary for sustaining the growth of prostate cancer epithelial cells in long-term tissue culture. Obviously, the "ideal" growth milieu has yet to be defined. Our laboratory is actively engaged in large-scale experiments to further enrich the in vitro growth environment. Additional factors that may enhance the growth of human prostate cancers in vitro include:

- Additional modifications in the basal nutrient medium, growth factors, or other additives
- Addition of exogenous TGF-α
- Use of mitogenic fractions of PC-3 CM and/or cancer stroma CM
- Incorporation of interleukin-6 (IL-6) to the growth milieu
- Addition of neutralizing TGF-β antibodies.

For example, we are currently testing a variety of alternative media formulations, one of which has been designated "complete" MEM, the constitution of which is described in table 2-2. It should be noted that MEM as a basal medium contains 1.8 x 10^{-3} *M* calcium, which contrasts with a calcium concentration of 1.3 x 10^{-4} *M* in WJAC-404. In addition, the concentrations of EGF and BPE have been significantly increased, while cholera toxin has been deleted altogether. The latter change was prompted by recent observations that cellular "euthanasia" may be mediated by

Table 2-2. Additives to MEM, an Alternative Media Formulation for the Growth of Prostate Epithelial Cells

"Complete" MEM Medium	
Fetal bovine serum	15%
Insulin	5 μg/ml
Transferrin	5 μg/ml
Selenous acid	5 ng/ml
Epidermal growth factor	20 ng/ml
Bovine pituitary extract	60 μg/ml
Prolactin	2.3 μg/ml
Dexamethasone	1×10^{-10} M
Dihydrotestosterone	1×10^{-10} M
Penicillin	100 U/ml
Streptomycin	100 μg/ml

increasing concentrations of nuclear ADP-ribosyl transferase. Cholera toxin ADP-ribosylates, the 45 kDa α-component of the stimulatory guanine nucleotide-binding protein of the adenyl cyclase system ($G_S\alpha$).[55] The latter event appears to reduce the affinity of $G_S\alpha$ for $Gi\beta$, which is a 35 kDa subunit of the inhibitory guanine nucleotide-binding protein that further inhibits adenyl cyclase activity when it interacts with the α subunit of G_S.[55] Indeed, some of the fresh prostate cancer targets tested in "complete" MEM appear to undergo more rapid proliferation and maintain a more compact morphology, with less tendency to develop dysplastic (senescent) features, after serial passage (figures 2-4A and 2-4B).

DHT has been deleted from other media preparations in the light of recent observations regarding the propensity of androgenic steroids to promote epithelial-fibroblastic conversion via syndecan gene suppression.[56] Syndecan is a cell-surface proteoglycan that serves as a matrix receptor and facilitates the anchorage of the cellular cytoskeleton to the extracellular matrix (ECM). Loss of syndecan expression could lead to decreased ECM recognition by prostate cancer cells in vitro with the subsequent induction of morphological and functional aberrations.

As noted previously, TGF-α appears to be an important mitogen involved in the autocrine/paracrine growth of the PC-3 tumor system.[41] The addition of exogenous TGF-α or TGF-α enriched fractions of PC-3 conditioned media to facilitate the growth

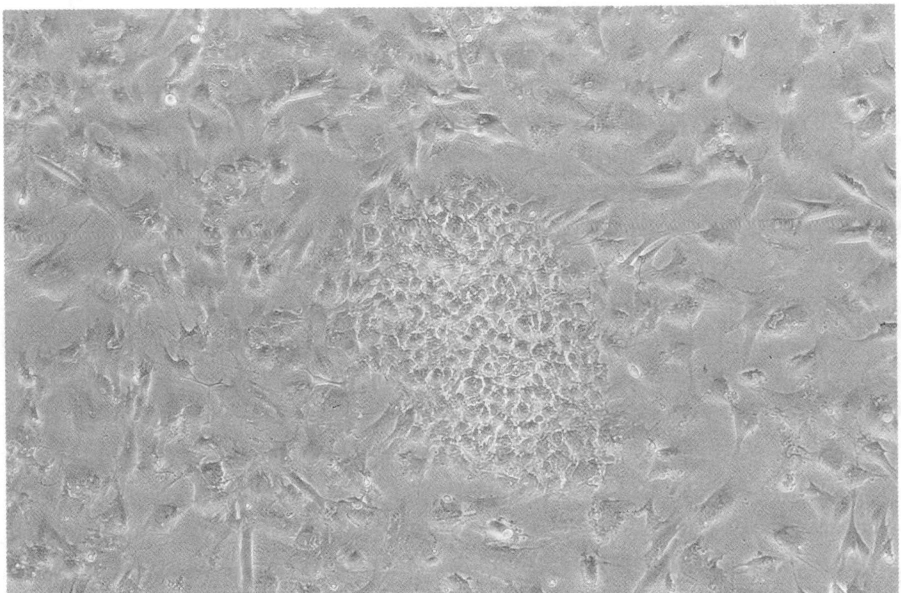

Figure 2-4A. Phase contrast micrograph of prostate cancer epithelial cells cultured on plastic in "complete" MEM. Cells maintain a more compact morphology over time.

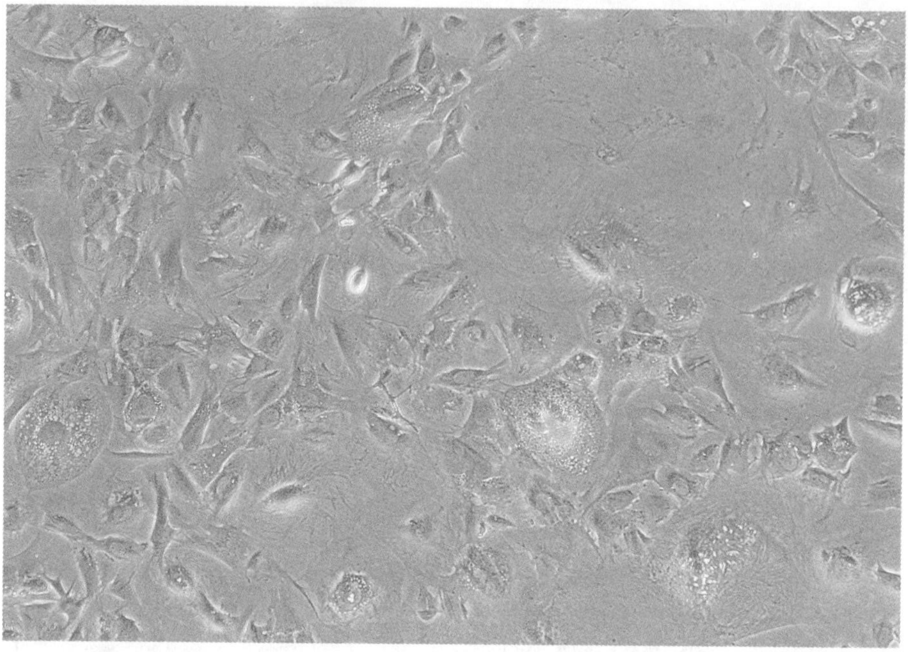

Figure 2-4B. Phase contrast micrograph of the same prostate cancer epithelial cells cultured on plastic in "complete" WAJC. Cells appear dysplastic and senescent.

of existing and fresh prostate systems in vitro is being aggressively tested at the present time (table 2-3). Along similar lines, our laboratory has demonstrated that the conditioned media from both BPH and cancer stromal cells is mitogenic for both BPH epithelial cells and prostate cancer targets, specifically PC-3 (figure 2-5). The isolation of highly mitogenic fractions from cancer stroma conditioned media is being pursued.

Table 2-3. Effect of TGF-α on Growth of Prostate Epithelial Cells In Vitro

	(Cell Number x 10^4)		
Group	**PC-3**	**DU-145**	**BPH Epithelial**
10% serum	125.3 ± 8.1	189.0 ± 9.6	120.0 ± 17.9
ITS	87.3 ± 6.6	32.0 ± 4.6	10.3 ± 1.7
TGF-α	102.5 ± 2.4	61.3 ± 9.4	64.0 ± 4.6

Cells were plated in 25 cm^2 tissue culture flasks and allowed to adhere overnight. The following day, plating media were replaced with RPMI-1640 medium containing 10% fetal bovine serum (positive control), ITS (negative control), or ITS plus TGF-α (10 ng/ml). Cultures were incubated for 6 days with media changes on days 2 and 4. On day 6, cells were detached by trypsinization and counted using a hemacytometer.

Interleukin-6 (IL-6) is a pleiotropic cytokine that has many reported functions, including (1) stimulation of activated B cells, (2) activity as a potent hepatocyte-stimulating factor, (3) hematopoietic factor, (4) a role in T cell activation, (5) neuronal differentiation, and (6) participation in IL-6/IL-6R autocrine loops in certain tumors.[57] With respect to the last issue, recent studies have demonstrated that PC-3, DU-145, and LNCaP produce IL-6 and express IL-6 receptors.[57] These observations suggest that the addition of exogenous IL-6 in vitro may facilitate the propagation of some fresh prostate cancer systems. This hypothesis is currently being tested in our laboratory.

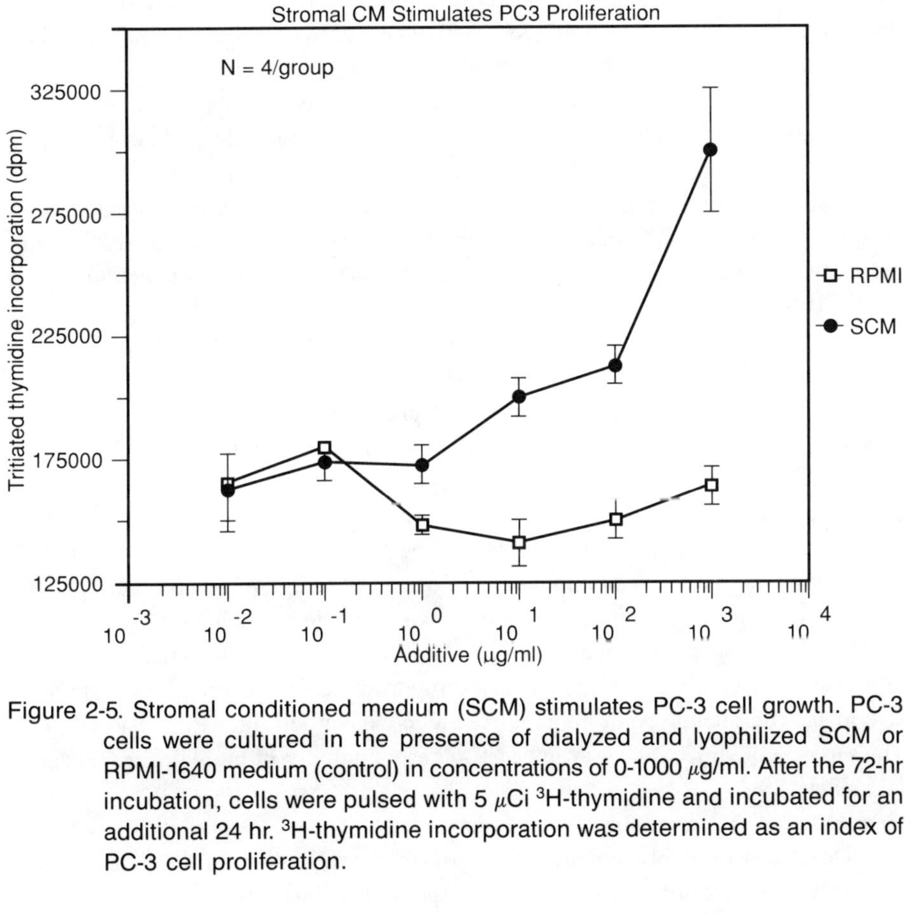

Figure 2-5. Stromal conditioned medium (SCM) stimulates PC-3 cell growth. PC-3 cells were cultured in the presence of dialyzed and lyophilized SCM or RPMI-1640 medium (control) in concentrations of 0-1000 μg/ml. After the 72-hr incubation, cells were pulsed with 5 μCi ^{3}H-thymidine and incubated for an additional 24 hr. ^{3}H-thymidine incorporation was determined as an index of PC-3 cell proliferation.

Finally, human breast cancer cells may induce negative autocrine regulation by the elaboration of transforming growth factor beta (TGF-β). This phenomenon can be abrogated by the addition of anti-TGF-β antibodies.[58] We are currently investigating whether the elaboration of TGF-β in prostate cancer systems is at least partly responsible for induction of the senescent phenotype and whether abrogation of its impact by neutralizing antibodies will facilitate in vitro growth.

Methods to Enhance In Vivo Propagation of Prostate Cancer Systems in Immune-Deficient Animals

In 1969, Rygaard and Povlsen first reported on the successful use of athymic nude mice for growing xenografted human tumors.[59] Despite the documented utility of this animal model for the study of many human tumors, this experimental system was thought to be of marginal value for the investigation of human prostate cancer. As stated previously, the successful xenografting of human prostate cancer in immune-deficient animals is a rare event. Moreover, immortalized prostate cancer cell lines derived from aggressive metastatic foci did not appear to exhibit conservation of their metastatic capacity when studied in nude mice.

Recent observations performed by ourselves and others have shown that the growth and metastasis of human prostate cancers implanted into nude mice is not a rare event.[28,36,60] In fact, this animal model has been used with great success with respect to the propagation, expansion, and in vivo selection of aggressive subpopulations existing within the PC-3 and DU-145 tumor systems.[28,36] These early studies suggested that the successful xenografting and subsequent metastasis of such tumors is more likely to occur:

- In animals with low levels of natural killer cell (NK-cell) activity
- By use of a large tumor inoculum (10^6-10^7 cells)
- Adoption of a prolonged experimental duration (8-12 wk)
- Supplementation of the gross examination of organs with a systematic search of likely target organs using appropriate histologic sections
- Planning the site of tumor injection in concert with the precepts of the cranial-caudal growth gradient, which favors the "craniad" deposition of tumor cells
- Inoculating tumor cells into more biologically "receptive" microenvironments, favoring orthotopic tumor deposition whenever feasible.[28]

These observations served as the catalyst for development of the intrasplenic injection assay.[28,36] The last approach appears to permit optimal expression of the invasive/metastatic phenotype of human prostate to cancer cell lines PC-3 and DU-145. The intrasplenic injection assay appears to have a number of biological advantages, including:

- Absence of a restrictive "pseudocapsule"
- Development of minimal tumor necrosis due to the enhanced vascularity of this injection site, somewhat akin to intraperitoneal injection
- Contingent on the cell line tested, can result in the production of tumor ascites
- Enhanced likelihood of tumor cell survival
- Direct access to the portal vein, providing a variant of the experimental metastasis assay
- Development of multifocal secondary metastases
- Adheres in principle to the cranial-caudal growth gradient.[28,36]

Table 2-4. Growth of Poorly Tumorigenic Prostate Cancer Cell Lines in Nude Mice

Cell line	Tumor formation – site of injection						
	A	B	C	D	E	F	G
	S.Q.−S	S.Q.+S	S.Q.−M	S.Q.+M	SRC−S	SRC+S	ISP
DU = 145	1/10	4/10	0/10	7/10	10/10	10/10	0/10
LNCaP	0/10	0/10	0/10	9/10	0/10	6/10	0/10

A = $1x10^6$ tumor cells in 0.2 ml PBS
B = $1x10^6$ tumor cells/$1x10^5$ prostate stromal cells in 0.2 ml PBS
C = $1x10^6$ tumor cells in 0.2 ml PBS
D = $1x10^6$ tumor cells in 0.1 ml PBS + 0.1 ml of reconstituted Matrigel
E = $1x10^6$ tumor cells in 0.1 ml PBS
F = $1x10^6$ tumor cells/$1x10^5$ prostate stromal cells in 0.1 ml PBS
G = $1x10^6$ tumor cells in 0.1 ml PBS

Despite the documented utility of the intrasplenic injection assay for the propagation and metastasis of the PC-3 tumor, cell line DU-145 is minimally tumorigenic and marginally metastatic when tested in this system. Moreover, the androgen-sensitive cell line LNCaP has not been successfully xenografted using this approach. Due to the fact that DU-145 and LNCaP are relatively refractory to facile growth in nude mice, we have used them as "targets" for a large series of experiments designed to enhance the utility of animal model systems for the maintenance of prostate cancer systems.

We have recently assessed a number of different approaches in the hope that such manipulation would facilitate the propagation of human prostate cancer in nude mice. The experimental approaches included:

- Varying the site of tumor injection to include intravenous (I.V.), subcutaneous (s.q.), subrenal capsule (SRC), and intrasplenic (ISP) routes
- Co-injection of tumor cells and "stromal" passengers
- Further alteration of the hormonal milieu by implanting time-release pellets containing DHT, 17-β estradiol, or 17-OH-progesterone
- Providing exogenous growth factors, such as TGF-α, EGF, or BPE
- Use of nude rats (T cell deficient) and SCID mice (T- and B cell deficient)
- Induction of further immune suppression in nude mice via splenectomy, cyclophosphamide administration, or antiasialo GM-1
- Co-injection of tumor cells with a basement membrane extracellular matrix (Matrigel).

The detailed results of these large-scale animal experiments will be reported elsewhere. However, it is possible to summarize some of the more interesting preliminary findings (table 2-4). When the site of tumor injection is the sole variable, the subrenal capsule deposition of suspension cells proves highly advantageous for the growth of DU-145. This route of injection provides tumor cells access to a highly vascularized environment containing TGF-α.[61] A caveat is required at this point, however. Unlike the subrenal capsule deposition of tumor fragments, injection of suspension cells—even in low volume—undoubtedly generates a substantial pressure within this enclosed space, possibly promoting parenchymal destruction and increasing the likelihood of cell-cell fusion. This may account for the relatively frequent observation of murine transformants noted on subsequent karyotypic analysis.

The injection of stromal "passengers" has been shown to augment the tumorigenic potential in a number of cell lines.[62] The exact mechanisms underlying this phenomenon are poorly understood, but they may relate to protection from host effector cells and beneficial stromal-epithelial signaling that may involve the elaboration of angiogenic growth factors. The subcutaneous growth of DU-145 and the SRC growth of cell line LNCaP was enhanced in the presence of stromal passengers. From a purely teleological standpoint, stromal-epithelial signaling events may be important in the evolution of both BPH and prostate cancer. Therefore, this observation in the animal model may have some relevance. To date, manipulation of the hormonal and growth factor environments appears to have little impact. However, the administration of time-released DHT pellets is probably advisable in order to avoid the circadian variation in circulating testosterone commonly noted in mice and rodents.[63] The intraperitoneal administration of TGF-α, EGF, and BPE did not appear to play a strategic role in enhancing local tumor growth. However, the use of more efficacious delivery vehicles (Alzet pumps) is being tested.

The athymic nude rat (rnu/rnu) was first observed in 1953.[64] Like the nude mouse (nu/nu), it possesses a rudimentary thymus and exhibits depressed or absent T cell function. Both animals, however, have intact B cell responses, normal macrophage activity, and amplified NK cell activity.[65] Theoretically, the nude rat possesses several distinct advantages. Its larger body size facilitates the conduct of manipulative procedures and serial blood sampling; in addition, it permits the orthotopic deposition of tumor material into the well-defined prostatic lobes.[66] In addition, the animal is more robust by nature and would require less stringent housing conditions. Finally, its life span of 1-2 yr permits long-term experimentation that would, theoretically, be of value in slow-growing tumor systems such as prostate cancers.

Numerous disadvantages of the nude rat include (1) a lower percentage of successful xenografts when compared to studies performed in nude mice, (2) a distinct propensity for growth followed by spontaneous regression, and (3) the infrequent documentation of tumor invasion and metastasis. We conducted pilot studies using the aggressive prostate cancer cell line PC-3 orthotopically injected into the ventral prostate of 6-wk-old male nude rats. Local tumor growth could be documented in host animals. However, the tumors never achieved large size, nor has metastasis occurred in the small number of animals tested to date.

Along similar lines, mice afflicted with the severe combined immune-deficiency syndrome (SCID mice) are intriguing given the fact that they are deficient in both T and B cell populations. Presumably, this enhanced degree of immunodeficiency would render them more receptive to human tumor xenografting. However, previous studies have not documented their overwhelming utility for the growth of genitourinary tumors.[67] More recently, we have documented the ability of these animals to support the growth of DU-145 and LNCaP when these tumor cells are injected in a Matrigel vehicle in subcutaneous sites. In this respect, however, they did not appear to be superior to nude mice of BALB origin.

As stated previously, Matrigel is a laminin-rich basement membrane biomatrix produced by the murine sarcoma, the Englebreth-Holm-Swarm (EHS) tumor that also contains type 4 collagen, heparan sulfate, and small amounts of entactin/nidogen.[18] In keeping with its biochemical constitution, this basement membrane preparation avidly sequesters heparan-binding growth factors, particularly basic fibroblast growth factor. It has recently been documented that co-injection of Matrigel and the poorly tumorigenic prostate cancer cell lines (DU-145, LNCaP) in subcutaneous sites greatly augments local tumor "take" and subsequent growth.[68] In fact, the studies of Fridman et al further validates these observations by demonstrating that Matrigel can enhance the tumorgenic potential in a number of nonprostatic murine and human tumor cell lines.[69] More recently, our laboratory has confirmed these observations and has documented that co-injection of these tumor cell lines with Matrigel (1:1) markedly augments the tumorigenicity of both cell lines. The beneficial impact of Matrigel with respect to the successful xenografting of these refractory human prostate cancer systems may be related to (1) a "protective" effect of the viscous basement membrane preparation vis-a-vis host effector cells and (2) the presence of angiogenic growth factors sequestered within the matrix, which could accelerate the neovascularization process at the critical incipient stage of tumor formation. As shown in figure 2-6, LNCaP tumor cell aggregates are surrounded by the "barrier" of Matrigel. Furthermore, an abundant amount of neovascularization is readily appreciated following analysis of histologic tumor sections. Additional studies have documented that the LNCaP xenografts heterogeneously express both PAP and PSA and secrete these markers into the peripheral blood from which they are detectable via radioimmunoassay.

Conclusion

From August 10, 1989, through April 9, 1991, our laboratory has acquired and processed 92 fresh prostate cancer tissues. Of these, 75 were derived from radical retropubic prostatectomy specimens, 14 from channel transuretheral resections, and 3 from metastatic sites. At this writing, 70% of the cancer specimens have been successfully adapted to in vitro growth and serial passage. To date, 28% of tumors propagated in vitro have been carried through >10 passages. In fact, 5 of the latter tumor systems have now achieved P levels in excess of 25. It should be emphasized that most of these tumors were of primary origin and were derived from low to intermediate Gleason histotype tumor systems. It is hoped that future improvements in

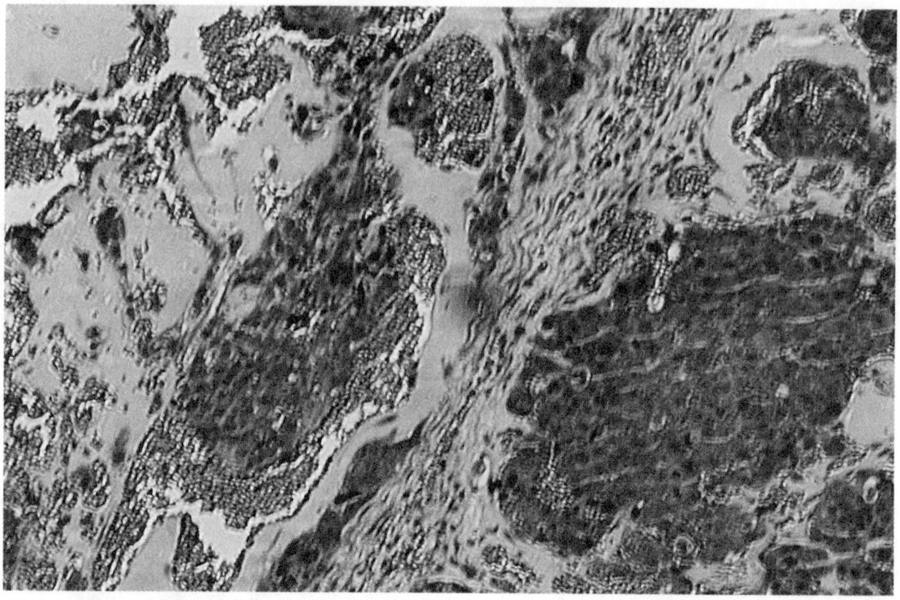

Figure 2-6. H&E stained section of an LNCaP tumor taken from nude mice. 1×10^6 tumor cells in 0.25 ml of Matrigel were deposited subcutaneously in the anterior aspect of the lateral thoracic region. Tumor growth was discernible after 3 wk. An abundant amount of neovascularization is observed in tumors co-injected with Matrigel.

our in vitro and in vivo methodology will permit the more routine cultivation of both androgen-sensitive and androgen-independent prostate cancers.

Finally, it should be emphasized that all newly established prostate cancer "systems" should be subjected to a rigorous battery of biologically relevant characterization studies. In our opinion, the latter should include:

- Growth curves
- Colony counts
- Plating efficiency
- Assessment of anchorage-independent growth in soft agar
- Construction of a cytokeratin profile
- Assessment of synthesis/secretion of PAP and PSA
- DNA flow cytometry
- 2-dimensional gel electrophoresis of whole cell extracts and conditioned medium
- Karyotype analysis
- Probing for nuclear androgen receptors
- Light/electron microscopy
- Growth in the nude mouse model.

Indeed, the ultimate utility of new prostate cancer systems will be reflected primarily by the biological information derived from such a multiphenotypic characterization.

References

1. Boring CC, Squires TS, Tong T. Cancer Statistics, 1991. CA 1991; 41:19-36
2. Kozlowski JM, Grayhack JT. Carcinoma of the prostate. In: Gillenwater JY, Grayhack JT, Howards SS, Duckett JW, eds. Adult and pediatric urology. vol 2. 2nd ed. St. Louis: Mosby Year Book, 1991; 1277-1393.
3. Grayhack JT, Keeler TC, Kozlowski JM. Carcinoma of the prostate: hormonal therapy. Cancer 1987; 60:(3 suppl):589-601.
4. Kozlowski JM, Ellis WJ, Grayhack JT. Advanced prostatic carcinoma—early versus late endocrine therapy. Urol Clin North Am 1991; 18:15-24.
5. Huggins C, Hodges CV. Studies on prostate cancer. I. The effect of castration, of estrogen, and of androgen injection on serum phosphatases in metastatic carcinoma of the prostate. Cancer Res 1941; 1:293.
6. McNeal JE. Normal histology of the prostate. Am J Surg Path Col 1988; 12:619-33.
7. McNeal JE, Price HM, Redwine EA, et al. Stage A versus stage B adenocarcinoma of the prostate: morphological comparison and biological significance. J Urol 1988; 139:61-5.
8. McNeal JE. The prostate gland: morphology and pathobiology. Monogr Urol 1983; 4:3-33.
9. Grayhack JT, Kozlowski JM. Benign prostatic hyperplasia. In: Gillenwater JY, Grayhack JT, Howards SS, Duckett JW, eds. Adult and pediatric urology. vol 2. 2nd ed. St. Louis: Mosby Year Book, 1991; 1211-76.
10. diSant'agnese PA, deMesy Jensen KL. Endocrine-paracrine cells of the prostate and prostatic urethra: an ultrastructural study. Hum Pathol 1984; 15:1034-41.
11. Hayashi N, Cunha GR, Wong YC. Influence of male genital tract mesenchymes on differentiation of Dunning prostatic adenocarcinoma. Cancer Res 1990; 50:4747-54.
12. Sherwood ER, Berg LA, McEwan RN, Pasciak RM, Kozlowski JM, Lee C. Two-dimensional protein profiles of cultured stromal and epithelial cells from hyperplastic human prostate. J Cell Biochem 1989; 40:201-14.
13. Sherwood ER, Berg LA, Mitchell NJ, Kozlowski JM, Lee C. Differential cytokeratin expression in normal, hyperplastic and malignant epithelial cells from human prostate. J Urol 1990; 143:167-71.
14. Brawer MK, Peehl DM, Stamey TA, Bostwick DG. Keratin immunoreactivity in the benign and neoplastic human prostate. Cancer Res 1985; 45:3663-7.
15. Isaacs JT, Coffey DS. Adaptation versus selection as the mechanism responsible for the relapse of prostatic cancer to androgen ablation therapy as studied in the Dunning R-3327-H adenocarcinoma. Cancer Res 1981; 41:5070-5.
16. Cunha GR, Donjacour AA, Cooke PS, et al. The endocrinology and developmental biology of the prostate. Endocr Rev 1987; 8:338-62.
17. Chung LWK, Cunha GR. Stromal-epithelial interactions. II. Regulation of prostatic growth by embryonic urogenital sinus mesenchyme. Prostate 1983; 4:503-11.
18. Kleinman HK, Klebe RJ, Martin GR. Role of collagenase matrices in the adhesion and growth of cells. J Cell Biol 1981; 88:473-85.
19. Rodriguez-Boulan E, Nelson WJ. Morphogenesis of the polarized epithelial cell phenotype. Science 1989; 245:718-24.
20. Bissel NJ, Hall GH, Parry G. How does the extracellular matrix direct gene expression? J Theor Biol 1982; 99:31-68.
21. Story MT, Sasse J, Jacobs SC, Lawson RK. Prostatic growth factor: purification and structural relationship to basic fibroblast growth factor. Biochemistry 1987; 26:3843-9.
22. Gospodarowicz D, Tauber JP. Growth factors in extracellular matrix. Endocrinol Rev 1980; 1:201.
23. Chung LWK, Chang SM, Bell C, Zhau H, Ro JY, von Eschenbach AC. Prostatic carcinogenesis evoked by cellular interaction. Environ Health Perspect 1988; 77:33-8.
24. Chung LWK, Chang S-M, Bell C, Zhau HE, Ro JY, von Eschenbach AC. Co-inoculation of tumorigenic rat prostate mesenchymal cells with nontumorigenic epithelial cells results in the development of carcinosarcoma in syngeneic and athymic animals. Int J Cancer 1989; 43:1179-87.

25. Noble RL. The development of prostatic adenocarcinoma in Nb rats following prolonged sex hormone administration. Cancer Res 1977; 37:1929-33.
26. Shain SA, McCullough B, Segaloff A. Spontaneous adenocarcinomas of the ventral prostate of aged AXC rats. JNCI 1975; 55:177-80.
27. Pollard M. Spontaneous prostate adenocarcinomas in aged germ-free Wistar rats. JNCI 1973; 51:1235-41.
28. Kozlowski JM, McEwan R, Keer H, et al. Prostate cancer and the invasive phenotype: application of new in vivo and in vitro approaches. In: Nicholson GL, Fidler IJ, eds. Tumor progression and metastasis. New York: AR Liss, 1988;189-231.
29. Kaighn ME, Shankar N, Ohnuki Y, Lechner JF, Jones LW. Establishment and characterization of a human prostatic carcinoma cell line (PC-3). Invest Urol 1979; 17:16-23.
30. Stone KR, Mickey DD, Wunderli H, Mickey GH, Paulson DF. Isolation of a human prostatic carcinoma cell line (DU-145). Int J Cancer 1978; 21:274-81.
31. Horoszewicz JS, Leong SS, Chu TM, et al. The LNCaP cell line - a new model for studies on human prostatic carcinoma. Prog Clin Biol Res 1980; 37:115-32.
32. Brothman AR, Lesho LJ, Somers KD, Wright GL Jr, Merchant DJ. Phenotypic and cytogenetic characterization of a cell line derived from primary prostatic carcinoma. Int J Cancer 1989; 44:898-903.
33. Schuurmans ALG, Bolt J, Mulder E. Androgen receptor-mediated growth and epidermal growth factor receptor induction in the human prostate cell line LNCaP. Urol Int 1989; 44:71-6.
34. Schuurmans ALG, Bolt J, Mulder E. Androgens stimulate both growth rate and epidermal growth factor receptor activity of the human prostate tumor cell LNCaP. Prostate 1988; 12:55-63.
35. Kozlowski JM, Sherwood ER, Fong C-J, Lee C. The impact of androgen, extracellular matrix, and stroma upon proliferation and differentiation of benign and malignant prostate epithelial cells. In: Coffey DS, Smith RG, Tindall DJ, Karr JP, eds. Molecular and cellular biology of prostate cancer, Prouts Neck, Maine, Oct 19-22, 1989. New York: Plenum Publishing (in press).
36. Kozlowski JM, Fidler IJ, Campbell D, Xu Z, Kaighn ME, Hart IR. Metastatic behavior of human tumor cell lines grown in the nude mouse. Cancer Res 1984; 44:3522-9.
37. Gaylis FD, Keer HN, Wilson J, Kwaan HC, Sinha AA, Kozlowski JM. Plasminogen activators in human prostate cancer cell lines and tumors: correlation with aggressive phenotype. J Urol 1989; 142:193-8.
38. Keer HN, Kozlowski JM, Tsai YC, Lee C, McEwan RN, Grayhack JT. Elevated transferrin receptor content in human prostate cancer cell lines assessed in vitro and in vivo. J Urol 1990; 143:381-5.
39. Hoehn W, Shroeder FH, Riemann JF, Joebsis AC, Hermanek P. Human prostatic adenocarcinoma, some characteristics of a serially transplantable line in nude mice (PC-82). Prostate 1980; 1:95-104.
40. Ito YZ, Nakazato Y. A new serially transplantable human prostatic cancer (HONDA) in nude mice. J Urol 1984; 132:384.
41. Hofer DR, Sherwood ER, Bromberg WD, Mendelsohn J, Lee C, Kozlowski JM. Autonomous growth of androgen-independent human prostatic carcinoma cells: role of transforming growth factor α. Cancer Res 1991; 51:2780-5.
42. Albini A, Iwamoto Y, Kleinman HK, et al. A rapid in vitro assay for quantitating the invasive potential of tumor cells. Cancer Res 1987; 47:3239-45.
43. Fong CY, Sherwood ER, Abu-Jawdeh GM, Kozlowski JM, Lee C. Reconstituted basement membrane promotes morphological and functional differentiation of primary prostatic epithelial cells (in press).
44. Ahmann FR, Woo L, Hendrix M, Trent JM. Growth in semisolid agar of prostate cancer cells obtained from bone marrow aspirates. Cancer Res 1986; 46:3560-4.
45. Mansi JL, Berger U, Wilson P, Shearer R, Coombes RC. Detection of tumor cells in bone marrow of patients with prostatic carcinoma by immunocytochemical techniques. J Urol 1988; 139:545-8.
46. Merchant DJ, Clarke SM, Ives K, Harris S. Primary explant culture: an in vitro model of the human prostate. Prostate 1983; 4:523-42.
47. Freeman AE, Hoffman RM. In vivo-like growth of human tumors in vitro. Proc Natl Acad Sci 1986; 83:2694-8.
48. Chaproniere DM, McKeenhan WL. Serial culture of single adult human prostatic epithelial cells in serum-free medium containing low calcium and a new growth factor from bovine brain. Cancer Res 1986; 46:819-24.

49. McKeehan WL, Adams PS, Rosser MP. Direct mitogenic effects of insulin, epidermal growth factor, glucocorticoid, cholera toxin, unknown pituitary factors and possibly prolactin, but not androgen, normal rat prostate epithelial cells in serum-free, primary cell culture. Cancer Res 1984; 44:1998-2010.
50. Kaighn ME. Human prostatic cells in serum-free medium. In: Fischer G, Wieser RJ, eds. Hormonally defined media. A tool in cell biology. First European Conference on Serum-Free Culture. Heidelberg: Springer-Verlag 1983;418-29.
51. Peehl DM, Stamey TA. Serial propagation of adult human prostatic epithelial cells with cholera toxin. In Vitro Cell Dev Biol 1984; 20:981-6.
52. Crabb JW, Armes LG, Johnson CM, McKeehan WL. Characterization of multiple forms of prostatropin (prostate epithelial cell growth factor) from bovine brain. Biochem Biophys Res Comm 1986; 136:1155-61.
53. Crabb JW, Armes LG, Karr SA, Johnson CM, Roberts GD, Bordoli RS, McKeehan WL. Complete primary structure of prostatropin, a prostate epithelial cell growth factor. Biochemistry 1986; 25:4988-93.
54. McKeehan WL, Adams PS. Heparan binding growth factor/prostatropin attenuate inhibition of rat prostate tumor epithelial cell growth by transforming growth factor type β. In Vitro Cell Dev Biol 1988; 24(3,part 1):243-6.
55. Gaal JC, Pearson CK. Covalent modification of proteins by ADP-ribosylation. TIBS 1986; 11:171-5.
56. Leppa SP, Harkonen P, Jalkanen N. Steroid-induced epithelial-fibroblastic conversion associated with syndecan suppression in S115 mouse mammary tumor cells. Cell Regulation 1991; 2:1-11.
57. Siegall CB, Schwab G, Nordan RP, Fitzgerald DJ, Pastan I. Expression of the interleukin-6 receptor and interleukin-6 in prostate carcinoma cells. Cancer Res 1990; 50:7786-8.
58. Arteaga CL, Coffey RJ Jr, Dugger TC, McCutchen CM, Moses HL, Lyons RM. Growth stimulation of human breast cancer cells with anti-transforming growth factor β antibodies: evidence for negative autocrine regulation by transforming growth factor β. Cell Growth Diff 1990; 1:367-74.
59. Rygaard J, Povlsen CO. Heterotransplantation of a human malignant tumor to nude mice. Acta Pathol Microbiol Scand 1969; A77:758-60.
60. Ware JL, Lieberman AP, Webb KS, Vollmer RT. Factors influencing phenotypic diversity of human prostate carcinoma cells metastasizing in athymic nude mice. Exp Cell Biol 1985; 53:163.
61. Gomella LG, Sargent ER, Wade TP, Anglard P, Linehan WM, Kasid A. Expression of transforming growth factor α in normal human adult kidney and enhanced expression of transforming growth factor α and $\beta 1$ in renal cell carcinoma. Cancer Res 1989; 49:6972-5.
62. Picard O, Rolland Y, Poupon MS. Fibroblast-dependent tumorigenicity of cells in nude mice: implication for implantation of metastases. Cancer Res 1986; 46:3290-4.
63. Kalra PS, Kalra SP. Circadian periodicities of serum androgens, progesterones, gonadotropins, and luteinizing hormone-releasing hormone in male rat: the effects of hypothalmic deafferentation, castration, and adrenalectomy. Endocrinology 1977; 101:1821.
64. Sawada M, Matsui Y, Hayakawa K, Nishiura H, Okudaira Y, Taki I. Human gynecologic cancers heterotransplanted into athymic nude rats. Gynecol Oncol 1982; 13:220-8.
65. Dejong WH, Steerenberg PA, Ursem PS, Osterhaus DME, Foss JG, Ruitenberg EJ. The athymic nude rat. III. Natural cell-mediated cytotoxicity. Clin Immunol Immunopathol 1980; 17:163-72.
66. Lee C. Gross dissection of three lobes of the rat prostate. Prog Clin Biol Res 1987; 239:577-82.
67. Phillips RA, Jewett MAS, Gallie BL. Growth of human tumors in a medium-deficient SCID mice and nude mice. Curr Top Microbiol Immunol 1989; 152:259-63.
68. Delmoro CM, Guckenberger GE, Pretlow TG. Human prostate carcinomas have increased tumorigenicity with Matrigel. FASEB abstr #5160, 1991.
69. Fridman R, Kibbey MC, Royce LS, et al. Enhanced tumor growth of both primary and established human and murine tumor cells in athymic mice after co-injection with Matrigel. JNCI 1991; 83:769-74.

3

THE USE OF TRANSRECTAL ULTRASOUND IN THE DIAGNOSIS OF PROSTATE CANCER

Martin I. Resnick, M.D.

Introduction

THE LACK OF PROGRESS in reducing the mortality rate from prostate cancer and the high proportion of patients with advanced disease at time of diagnosis makes screening and early diagnosis a seemingly efficacious and desirable endeavor. If the percentage of men whose tumors are localized and diagnosed could be increased, it is reasonable to assume that the mortality rate could be lowered. Asymptomatic patients with localized prostate cancer can potentially be cured with either radical prostatectomy or radiation therapy. Given these considerations, early detection and treatment of prostate cancer may therefore seem to be a logical step in reducing mortality from this disease; however, no controlled studies have proved that screening for prostate cancer by any method is able to accomplish this goal.

The rapid development of transrectal ultrasound has resulted in considerable enthusiasm for its use as a screening test for early detection of prostate cancer, but most reports advocating transrectal ultrasound for this purpose have been "case finding" studies and not controlled clinical trials. Lee et al reported transrectal ultrasound to be twice as sensitive as digital rectal examination in screening 784 men over 60 for prostate cancer, with detection rates of 2.6 and 1.3 percent, respectively.[1]

It must be emphasized that because 50% of the men had a normal digital rectal examination within 1 yr prior to the study, the number of biopsies performed for an abnormal digital rectal examination would be expected to be diminished; indeed, the biopsy rate was twice as high based on transrectal ultrasound indications as compared to digital rectal examination indications. It can, therefore, be concluded that the increased biopsy rate alone may have been responsible for the increased cancer detection rate with use of transrectal ultrasound. Studies have in fact demonstrated that blind biopsies on patients with palpably benign prostates have a reported cancer detection rate as high as 4%.[2] Another important concept regarding the study is to recognize that because the ultrasound criteria for biopsy included only patients with hypoechoic lesions in the peripheral zone of the gland, a substantial number of cancers may have been missed among the 707 patients with normal ultrasound examinations who did not undergo biopsy. Comparisons between ultrasound examinations and corresponding whole-mount histologic specimens of radical prostatectomy specimens have demonstrated that 25-30% of prostate cancers are isoechoic and are not visualized with ultrasound.[3] Studies also have shown that although 40% of cancers arise anterior to the midportion of the prostate in the transverse plane and are nonpalpable, these cancers are also the most difficult to detect with current ultrasound imaging techniques. Additionally, large diffuse tumors often cannot be clearly differentiated from surrounding nonmalignant tissue with ultrasound; predictably, the 2 largest tumors from the Lee series were diagnosed with digital rectal examination alone and were not visualized on the initial ultrasound examination.

Effect of Improved Screening Methods

A recent report by Cooner et al revealed that the overall rate of prostate cancer detection from screening could be significantly increased from 1.7% with the use of digital rectal examination alone to 14.6% with the combined use of digital rectal examination, serum prostatic specific antigen determination, and transrectal ultrasonography.[4] In order to achieve this high detection rate, about half of the patients presenting for evaluation underwent prostatic biopsy. Data collected by the Cooner group also indicate that if a patient has a negative digital rectal examination and a prostatic-specific antigen level within the normal range, the chance of carcinoma of the prostate being present is unlikely, even in the presence of an abnormal ultrasound study. Although the authors recommend that all men over 65 have a prostate ultrasound examination, they believe that younger men should have the study only if either the digital rectal examination and/or the prostatic-specific antigen determination is abnormal.

Although studies using digital rectal examination to screen for prostate cancer have been limited, cancer detection rates of 0.8-1.6% have been reported.[5] Using this method, detection studies have also determined that screened patients have been found to have lower clinical stage cancers than are found in unscreened patients, fewer cancers at subsequent follow-up visits, and lower clinical and pathological stage of detected cancers if a previous digital rectal examination had been negative.[6] Although detection of prostate cancer with digital rectal examination may not be ideal, several advantages are apparent. It is inexpensive, usually requiring less than 5 min, and can be easily incorporated into a routine physical examination performed by all physicians that would also allow for the assessment and/or detection of other diseases as well. Although a significant number of patients with palpably localized prostate cancer will be upstaged pathologically, using the previous argument regarding "clinical" significance, one may speculate that the larger lesions detected by digital rectal examination are of higher biological potential and more threatening to the patient than the small lesions detected by other means.

As with most aspects of health care in the 1990s, the cost of screening for prostate cancer by any method warrants careful evaluation. At $150 per examination, it would cost $3.75 million to perform one transrectal ultrasound study on the 25 million American men over 50. Assuming a 10% biopsy rate, at $160 per biopsy, an additional $400 million would be needed, bringing the total cost to $4.1 billion. If it is assumed (1) that at lease 30% of men over 50 harbor prostate cancer and (2) that the overall detection rate for transrectal ultrasound is 3%, $4.1 billion would be spent for detecting 10% of all prostate cancers, the potential clinical significance of which is unknown. While variable, the cost of digital rectal examination is most certainly less than that of transrectal ultrasound, and the biopsy rate with digital examination most likely would be less than it would be with transrectal ultrasound. Whether the 2 studies are equivalent regarding patient outcome (i.e., mortality) is unknown. A recent report analyzing the economics of prostate cancer screening concludes that the cost of such a program in men between the ages of 50-70 would be prohibitive.[7]

Improved Survival Not Yet Demonstrated

While the detection of lower stage disease at time of diagnosis may result from routine screening procedures for prostate cancer, the procedure of choice in terms of patient survival has yet to be determined. Therefore, screening for prostate cancer with ultrasound cannot be advocated at this time because the potential benefits related to early detection have not been demonstrated to outweigh the potential risks related to the morbidity and mortality associated with increased diagnosis and treatment. More important, as already noted, it has not yet been demonstrated that a screened population has reduced mortality when compared to an unscreened population. A large prospective, controlled screening trial is now being planned by the National Cancer Institute in which patients will be randomized to a screened or control (unscreened) population. Screened patients of a standardized age range (i.e., 60-74 yr) will be subjected to standardized tests (e.g., digital rectal examination, prostatic-specific antigen, transrectal ultrasonography) performed at specified times and intervals (e.g., yearly) and unscreened patients will be cared for and evaluated in a non-prescribed manner, thus representing the general population. Treatment will be instituted based on disease stage at time of diagnosis, and all patients will be followed, with specific prostate cancer mortality being the end point. This comparative study not only will demonstrate the benefit or lack of benefit of screening but should also identify the optimum method of screening, the optimum time interval for screening, and the optimal patient population to be screened. Until this study is completed, transrectal ultrasound cannot be considered a legitimate screening examination for the early detection and diagnosis of prostate cancer.

References

1. Lee F, Littrup PJ, Torp-Pederson ST, et al. Prostate cancer: comparison of transrectal ultrasound and digital rectal examination for screening. Radiology 1989; 168:389.
2. Agasteon EH, Hernandez FJ, Layfield FJ. The use of fine needle aspiration for the detection of stage A prostate carcinoma before transurethral resection of the prostate: a clinical trial. J Urol 1987; 138:551.
3. Shinohara K, Wheeler TM, Scardino PT. The appearance of prostate cancer on transrectal ultrasonography: correlation of imaging of pathological examinations. J Urol 1989; 142:76.
4. Cooner WH, Mosley BR, Rutherford CL Jr, et al. Prostate cancer detection in a clinical urological practice by ultrasonography, digital rectal examination and prostatic specific antigen. J Urol 1990; 143:1146.
5. Chodak GW, Schoenberg HW. Progress and problems in screening for carcinoma of the prostate. World J Surg 1989; 13:60.
6. Thompson IM, Farr WR. Screening for carcinoma of the prostate: efficacy of available screening tests. World J Surg 1989; 13:65.
7. Optenberg SA, Thompson IM. Economics of screening for carcinoma of the prostate. Urol Clin North Am 1990; 17:719.

4

PATIENT SELECTION FOR RADICAL PROSTATECTOMY

William J. Catalona, M.D.

THE MOST APPROPRIATE CANDIDATES for radical prostatectomy are patients with clinically organ-confined prostate cancer who are in good general health and have a life expectancy of at least 10 yr. Some authors have advocated radical prostatectomy for selected patients with locally advanced disease (stage C1) and some with limited regional lymph node metastases (stage D1); however, there is no convincing evidence to support a *curative* role for radical prostatectomy in patients with extracapsular tumor extension. Furthermore, no convincing data support the notion that prophylactic radical prostatectomy in patients with extracapsular tumor extension confers any therapeutic benefits other than a possible temporary psychological boost to the patient and his family.

Status of Potency-Sparing Surgery

There is accumulating evidence that more restrictive selection criteria should be used for potency-sparing radical prostatectomy; (1, 3) however, at the present the indications for this operation have not yet been clearly defined. Potency-sparing radical prostatectomy has 2 separate and sometimes mutually exclusive objectives: (1) complete tumor excision and (2) preservation of the neurovascular bundles responsible for erectile potency. The potency-sparing operation requires that the surgeon perform the dissection in a plane immediately adjacent to the prostatic capsule in order to spare the neurovascular bundles.[4] With this operation, potency can be preserved in most patients.[1,5] Moreover, the operation can be modified so that the neurovascular bundles can be widely excised in patients found to have extracapsular tumor extension at time of operation.[6]

Questions have arisen about whether the potency-sparing operation compromises the classical principles of cancer surgery.[1,3] In an early histopathological study of 100 consecutive nerve-sparing radical prostatectomy specimens, Eggleston and Walsh reported that 41% had capsular penetration of tumor and only 7% had positive surgical margins.[6] In none of these patients were the margins positive only at the site of the nerve-sparing modification. In contrast, Stamey et al reported that in the great majority of patients with extracapsular tumor extension, the extension occurred in the area of the ipsilateral neurovascular bundle.[2] More recently, Stamey suggested that the apical dissection as described by Walsh in the nerve-sparing radical prostatectomy compromises the apical surgical margins.[3] Stamey recommended that the nerve-sparing operation should *not* be attempted in patients having an apical nodule,[3] and that only unilateral nerve-sparing should be attempted in patients having a unilateral nodule.[2]

Our results suggest that patients having focal, well-differentiated tumors—i.e., patients with clinical stages A1 and B1 or B2 tumors—are the most suitable candidates for the nerve-sparing radical prostatectomy.[1] Those with bulky, diffuse, and/or poorly-differentiated tumors are not good candidates for nerve-sparing because they have a high incidence of microscopic extracapsular tumor penetration, often at the apex or in the region of the neurovascular bundles. In our experience, although potency was preserved overall in 63% of patients who underwent bilateral nerve-sparing operations, simultaneous complete tumor excision and preservation of potency was achieved in 71% of clinical stage A1 patients, 39% of clinical stage A2 patients, 56% of clinical stage B1 patients, and only 24% of clinical stage B2 patients.

Benefits of Wider Dissection Unclear

Although theoretically it seems logical to assume that patients who have wider dissections will have a lower incidence of positive margins, it has not yet been definitely proven that a higher percentage of these patients can be rendered tumor-free by wider dissection. Furthermore, the anticipated therapeutic benefits of resecting the neurovascular bundles in patients with extracapsular tumor extension have not yet been formally demonstrated.

We have been unable to predict accurately at time of operation which patients have microscopic extracapsular tumor extension and which have periprostatic fibrosis. For example, among patients who had both neurovascular bundles sacrificed for presumed tumor extension, 38% were found to have histologically organ-confined tumors. Similarly, 45% of patients who had one neurovascular bundle sacrificed were also found to have completely organ-confined tumors. On the other hand, in patients who had both neurovascular bundles preserved because the tumor appeared to be totally encapsulated at the time of operation, 38% were found to have extracapsular tumor extension on histological examination of the specimen. Thus, errors were commonly made in both directions.

Summary

In summary, patients with clinical stage A and B prostate cancer are legitimate candidates for radical prostatectomy. Alternatively, patients with clinical A1 disease may be followed conservatively with serial PSA levels, although younger patients will be at greater risk of disease progression than older patients. The nerve-sparing operation is appropriate for selected patients with low or intermediate grade, low-volume stage A1 and B1 tumors and some patients with small stage B2 tumors. The standard radical prostatectomy is more appropriate for patients with high-volume and poorly differentiated stage A2 and large B2 tumors. Although it seems logical to expect greater cure rates with the standard radical prostatectomy than the nerve-sparing radical prostatectomy, this has not yet been formally demonstrated.

References

1. Catalona WJ, Bigg SW. Nerve-sparing radical prostatectomy: evaluation of results after 250 patients. J Urol 1990; 143:538.
2. Stamey TA, McNeal JE, Freiha FS, Redwine E. Morphometric and clinical studies on 68 consecutive radical prostatectomies. J Urol 1988; 138:1235.
3. Stamey TA, Villers AA, McNeal JE, Link PC, Freiha FS. Positive surgical margins at radical prostatectomy: importance of the apical dissection. J Urol 1990; 143:1166.
4. Walsh PC. Radical retropubic prostatectomy. In: Walsh PC, Gittes RF, Perlmutter AD, et al, eds. Campbell's textbook of urology, 5th ed. Philadelphia: W.B. Saunders, 1986.
5. Walsh PC. Radical prostatectomy, preservation of sexual function, cancer control: the controversy. Urol Clin North Am 1987; 14:633.
6. Eggleston JC, Walsh PC. Radical prostatectomy with preservation of sexual function: pathologic findings in the first 100 cases. J Urol 1985; 134:1146.

5

CONTROVERSIES IN RADIATION THERAPY IN THE MANAGEMENT OF PROSTATE TUMORS

Ramananda M. Shetty, M.D.

Introduction

RADIATION HAS BEEN USED in treating prostate carcinoma since early in this century. In 1911, Pasteau published his experience of successfully treating a physician with prostate carcinoma with a series of insertions of a rubber catheter containing radium sources.[1] The real breakthrough in the role of radiation in the management of prostate carcinoma came in the 1960s when Bagshaw et al[2] and Budhraja and Anderson[3] published their experience of treating these tumors with megavoltage radiation and showed that prostate cancer can, indeed, be effectively treated with radiation with an acceptable level of complications.

One of the major unsettled controversies is the role of adjuvant radiation therapy in the management of pathologic stage C adenocarcinoma of the prostate. Anywhere from 30% to 50% of patients with Stage A and B adenocarcinoma of the prostate who have undergone radical prostatectomy are found to have pathologic state C tumor. The tumor is found outside the gland, involving the seminal vesicle, surgical margin, or adjacent organs. There is no unanimous agreement among urologists and radiation oncologists about the management of pathologic stage C carcinoma of the prostate. There is the prevailing impression among some urologists that when tumors are outside the capsule, the majority of them are bound to fail distantly and adjuvant radiation to the pelvis is not beneficial.[4,5] On the other hand, the majority of radiation oncologists feel that these patients are not only high-risk candidates for distant spread but also equally high-risk candidates for local failure, and that by controlling the local failure with immediate postoperative radiation, long-term survival also probably can be improved.[5-7]

Northwestern University Experience

From 1975 to 1976, 73 patients who underwent radical prostatectomy for stage A and B carcinoma of the prostate were found to have tumor outside the prostatic capsule at the surgical margin, seminal vesicle, or in the adjacent organ.[4] Out of 73, only 16 were referred to radiation and all received postoperative radiation either to the prostate bed or to the whole pelvis. The dose range was 4,500-7,200 cGy in 5-8 wk. Out of the 16, 8 also had microscopic lymph node involvement (Stage D1). The median follow-up of these patients is 65 mo, and the range of follow-up is 25-125 mo. All 16 irradiated patients are free from local recurrence (100%), whereas 11/56 (19%) of the patients who did not receive postoperative radiation developed local recurrence. Although disease-free survival is superior with the radiation group, the difference between these 2 groups has not achieved statistical significance at this time.

Gibbons et al of Mason Clinic, Seattle, irradiated 22 of 45 patients with pathologic stage C carcinoma after perineal prostatectomy.[7] The radiation dose range was 4,900-7,200 cGy, with an average dose of 6,325 cGy. Of the 23 who did not receive postoperative radiation, 30% recurred locally, whereas only 1/22 irradiated patients (5%) failed locally. Distant failure only was 35% for nonirradiated and 23% for the irradiated group. Of the group of 45, 59% of the irradiated patients and 35% of the nonirradiated patients are alive without disease at a mean follow-up of 9.2 yr.

Gordon et al of Stanford University treated 13 patients for extracapsular extension with postoperative irradiation with a dose ranging from 5,500 to 6,600 cGy; they reported a 5- to 10-yr disease-free survival of 57%.[8]

It is a well-accepted fact that radiation controls local recurrence effectively, but the controversy has not been settled over whether it will improve long-term survival. Currently, the Southwest Oncology Group has embarked on a study of randomizing pathologic stage C patients either to an observation arm or to adjuvant radiation therapy. It is hoped that this study will end the controversy once and for all.

References

1. Pasteau O. Traitement du cancer de la prostate par le radium. Revue des Maladies de la Nutrition, 1911.
2. Bagshaw MA, Kaplan HS. Radical external radiation therapy of localized prostate carcinoma. Proc 10th Intl Cong Radiol. Montreal, Canada, Sept 1962.
3. Budhraja SN, Anderson JC. An assessment of the value of radiotherapy in the management of carcinoma of the prostate. Br J Urol 1964; 36:535-40.
4. Smith JA SR, Middleton RG. Clinical management of prostate cancer. Chicago: Yearbook Medical Publishers, 1987.

5. Paulson DF et al. Postoperative radiotherapy of the prostate for patients undergoing radical prostatectomy with positive margins, seminal vesicle involvement and/or penetration through the capsule. J Urol 1970; 143:1178-92.
6. Shevlin BE et al. The role of adjuvant irradiation following primary prostatectomy, based on histopathologic extent of tumor Int J Radiat Oncol Biol, Phys 16: 1425-30, 1989.
7. Gibbons RP et al. Adjuvant radiotherapy following radical prostatectomy: results and complications. J Urol 1986; 135:65-68.
8. Ray GR, Bagshaw MA, Freiha F. External beam radiation salvage for residual or recurrent local tumor following radical prostatectomy. J Urol 1984; 132:926-30.

6

OVERVIEW OF HORMONAL THERAPY IN PROSTATE CANCER

John T. Grayhack, M.D.

Background

"IN MANY INSTANCES THE malignant prostatic tumor is an overgrowth of adult epithelial cells. All known types of prostatic epithelium undergo atrophy when androgenic hormones are greatly reduced in amount or inactivated. In this paper, evidence is presented that significant improvement often occurs in the clinical condition of patients with far advanced cancer of the prostate after they have been subjected to castration."

This introductory paragraph to the 1941 manuscript by Huggins et al reporting the initiation of hormonal therapy of carcinoma of the prostate summarized the rationale for this therapeutic approach. The data presented represented a landmark leap in the treatment of malignancy because they demonstrated the effectiveness of a systemic approach to the control of cancer. Two other facets of this contribution to our care of patients are important: (1) the use of systemic markers to evaluate and monitor the status of malignancy was introduced, and (2) the observations that led Huggins and his associates to propose and carry out orchiectomy were based on laboratory investigations. As sex steroids and gonadotropins became available, the Huggins group began to explore their effects on prostatic physiology, using the dog prostatic fistula model that had been developed initially by Dr. Farrell of Northwestern University. Observations on the effects of androgen withdrawal and administration on the growth and function of the dog prostate reinforced the evidence of the rapid, profound changes that could be induced in the prostatic cells by hormonal manipulation. At about the same time, Kutcher and Wolbergs and the Gutmans demonstrated that normal prostatic epithelial cells had an extremely high concentration of acid phosphatase that persisted in malignancy. Furthermore, the serum level of acid phosphatase was demonstrated to be increased in men with metastatic carcinoma of the prostate as compared with the level in disease-free men. These observations, combined with other supportive data, provided the critical preliminary information that led to the employment of orchiectomy and estrogen to treat patients with advanced metastatic cancer of the prostate.

Primary Factors in Hormonal Manipulation

Several important aspects of hormonal manipulation in patients with prostate carcinoma warrant emphasis. The clinically identifiable response rate to orchiectomy or an alternative therapy is undoubtedly dependent on the parameters used to measure response, such as prostatic induration and volume, serum acid phosphatase and prostate-specific antigen, and soft-tissue and bone changes. Clinical response rates varying from 60% to 80% of patients treated have been reported. As indicators of response become more sensitive, observed rates may well increase without any real change in actual response. The likelihood that none of the malignant cells derived from a prostatic acinar or ductal source would be androgen-dependent seems limited. This prejudice is reaffirmed by the observed evidence of increased tumor activity in patients with carcinoma of the prostate who have been given exogenous androgen. The Huggins group administered androgen to 3 patients with metastatic disease and demonstrated a prompt response of carcinoma of the prostate manifested both by an increase in acid phosphatase levels and bone pain. Others have confirmed and expanded on this observation. Fowler and Whitmore reported that 45-55 patients with metastatic prostate carcinoma who had an evaluable response after exogenous testosterone administration developed evidence of progressive disease. Only 4 of these patients had received no previous endocrine therapy; 34 had symptomatic relapse after endocrine manipulation, and 14 were in symptomatic endocrine-induced remission. The Fowler and Whitmore observations and those of others indicated that not only the previously untreated tumor but also the malignancy in patients who had undergone androgen withdrawal procedures for prolonged periods maintains the capacity to be stimulated by exogenous androgen. These observations clearly argue against unmonitored discontinuance of androgen-suppressive measures, even when recurrent tumor activity occurs in their presence. Additionally, it seems highly probable that the discordance between the identified and expected incidence of tumor response to increased androgen levels that may occur transiently after unmodified LH-RH administration is related to the insensitivity of monitoring procedures.

The response to orchiectomy of patients with metastatic prostatic carcinoma is often rapid and dramatic. Relief of severe bone pain can occur within hours after an orchiectomy performed under local anesthesia. Markedly elevated serum acid phosphatase or PSA levels may fall to normal within days. The rapid response to endocrine manipulation should make this approach the primary tumor-directed effort in patients with life- and organ-threatening disease (e.g., spinal cord involvement or ureteral obstruction). Androgen withdrawal should be initiated urgently and with precedent in this group of individuals.

The concept of possible persistent stimulation of some prostatic cancer cells by the very low levels of biologically active androgen secreted by the adrenals has been considered since shortly after the high initial response rate and subsequent recurrence of tumor activity following orchiectomy or estrogen administration was recognized. Objective evidence to support this possibility is the demonstrated persistence of low, but higher than expected, intracellular DHT levels in some tumors after orchiectomy or extrogen therapy and the minimal stimulation of the prostate that probably results from adrenal androgens in some selected circumstances in rodents. A variety of surgical procedures, including bilateral adrenalectomy with and without glucocorticoid replacement, unilateral adrenalectomy and hepatic shunting of left adrenal venous blood, and hyposectomy, have been used in an effort to eliminate adrenal androgens, but little convincing evidence of significant alteration in the patient's course has emerged. More recently, pharmacologic measures have been used to reevaluate this concept of "total androgen ablation." My own belief is that if these measures have any effect on survival, it is limited, and that with our limited resources, we would do well to concentrate our efforts on other approaches to the control of metastatic disease.

Timing of Hormone Therapy

The timing of initiation of hormone therapy has been controversial and remains so. No definite survival advantage can be demonstrated for prompt versus delayed initiation of hormonal manipulation in a clinical setting. This contrasts with some evidence suggesting that early initiation of hormone therapy is advantageous in animal models used to study prostatic carcinoma. The complexity of the clinical circumstances may well hamper identification of differences in progression and survival related to the tumor when therapy is initiated promptly on diagnosis as compared to delayed therapeutic intervention even if these exist.

Clinical observations of patients with advanced carcinoma of the prostate after orchiectomy or testis suppression have provided interesting information that tends to confirm observations made in more controlled settings. Urologists have long recognized that one focus of tumor such as the primary site will respond and remain quiescent throughout the patient's course while another either will not respond or will resume growth. Furthermore, comparison of grade and DNA ploidy in initial tumor biopsies as compared with biopsies of recurrent tumor after hormone therapy almost always demonstrate a grade and ploidy migration toward less differentiated cells. These observations provide clinical evidence to support the clonal differences in the cancer cell populations that are much more easily demonstrated in various laboratory settings. As has been noted before, the recurrence of the production of a presumably androgen-dependent secretory protein such as acid phosphatase or prostate-specific androgen in an androgen-deprived environment is a paradox that warrants recognition and evaluation. Equally interesting is the stimulation of these enzymes by administration of exogenous androgens in these circumstances.

Not all observations derived from patients subjected to hormonal manipulation relate directly to the carcinoma. Among these, the cardiovascular effects of pharmacologic amounts of female hormone, the development and control of hot flashes in patients subjected to orchiectomy and LH-RH administration, and the persistence of sexual function in elderly males subjected to androgen ablative measures have added to our knowledge and challenged our understanding of a variety of organ/system effects not directly related to the prostate. As we vary and expand our efforts with hormonal manipulation to alter the status of a patient's prostate cancer, we should be alert to other possible effects of these therapeutic endeavors.

Bibliography

1. Huggins C, Stevens RE Jr., Hodges CV. Studies in prostatic cancer. II. The effects of castration on advanced carcinoma of the prostate gland. Arch Surg 1941; 43:209.
2. Huggins C, Hodges CV. Studies in prostatic cancer. I. Effect of castration, of estrogen, and of androgen on serum phosphatases in metastatic carcinoma of prostate. Cancer Res 1941; 1:293.
3. Geller J, Albert JD, Nachtsheim DA, Loza 0. Comparison of prostatic cancer tissue dehydrotestosterone levels at the time of relapse following orchiectomy or estrogen therapy. J Urol 1984; 132:693.
4. Grayhack JT, Wendel EF. Hormone dependence of carcinoma of the prostate. In: E. Brandes, ed. Male accessory sex organs, structure and function in mammals. New York, San Francisco, London: Academic Press, 1974; 425.
5. Grayhack JT. Hormonal treatment of prostate cancer. Surg Clin North Am 1959; 39:13.
6. Grayhack JT, Keeler T, Kozlowski J. Carcinoma of the prostate: hormone therapy. Cancer 1987; 60:589.
7. Resnick MI, Grayhack, JT. Treatment of stage IV carcinoma of the prostate. Urol Clin North Am 1975; 2:141.
8. Walsh P. Physiologic basis in hormonal therapy in carcinoma of the prostate. Urol Clin North Am 1975; 2:125.

7

ROLE OF ANTIANDROGENS IN THE MANAGEMENT OF ADVANCED PROSTATE CANCER

E. David Crawford, M.D.

Introduction

TOTAL ANDROGEN SUPPRESSION REFERS to the employment of means to suppress the effect of adrenal as well as testicular androgens. Although the concept itself is not new, the emergence of new drugs previously described have rekindled interest. Protagonists point to the statistic that about 30% of patients with advanced prostate cancer who relapse with disease progression after traditional endocrine therapy respond to surgical and medical adrenalectomy. Additionally, it is recognized that in patients thought to be hormonal refractory, the administration of testosterone can result in disease exacerbation. Supporters of this approach argue that these findings signified continued hormonal responsiveness, and conclude that low levels of adrenal androgens contribute to the growth of prostate tumors.

Two theories exist to explain clinical relapse in patients treated with monotherapy only. These models of hormone resistance attempt to explain the phenomenon on the cellular level. The first theory is that prostate cancer cells are variably sensitive to androgens, and that relapse following initial successful treatment is the result of inadequate suppression of androgens, i.e., the adrenal component. According to this theory, total androgen blockade would produce a more profound reduction in hormonal clones and produce a prolonged time to progression and increased survival.

The second model proposes that cells are heterogeneous in their growth requirement for androgens, and that relapse is the result of the development of resistant clones. In this scenario, total androgen blockade would have little to no effect.

Findings in Animal Studies

Animal studies exist to support both theories. The principal model employed is the androgen-sensitive Shionogi mouse mammary cancer model. This model has been used both to support and refute the value of combined androgen blockade. In several studies, preincubation of the androgen-sensitive Shionogi mouse mammary cancer cells for 15 days in the absence of androgen results in the development of complete resistance of growth to the effect of androgens. However, androgen sensitivity was maintained by incubation with flutamide in the absence of androgens. This study implies that the administration of antiandrogens might avoid, or at least delay, the development of androgen resistance, thus improving the success of therapy.

Ellis and Isaacs have performed a series of experiments comparing the effects of partial versus complete androgen ablation in the treatment of rats with the Dunning 3327H (a well-differentiated tumor) and 3327R (a poorly differentiated tumor). Using control groups, tumor-bearing rats were treated with either orchiectomy alone or with orchiectomy and cyproterone acetate and a progestational antiandrogen. No difference in growth or survival was seen in the 2 groups.

Theoretical arguments aside, the definitive laboratory lies in the hospital ward. Investigators have designed studies evaluating the clinical response of patients with stage D2 prostate cancer, comparing combined therapy with monotherapy as the control. Labrie is the most strident advocate of the benefits of combined therapy. Unfortunately, his studies were not randomized and were from a single institution. Several studies have been performed with combined androgen blockade, and the results have been mixed. One of the larger studies, done by Beland et al in Canada, compared an LH-RH analogue and Anandron to an LH-RH analogue and a placebo. The group registered 211 patients, and the results revealed a statistically significant difference in progression-free survival and survival favoring the combined androgen blockade group. However, the combination therapy was significantly more toxic than monotherapy.

National Cancer Institute Study

The largest study ever performed in advanced prostate cancer was begun in 1984, sponsored by the National Cancer Institute. This study was designed to evaluate the possible benefit for combined androgen therapy. The design was placebo-controlled, double-blind, prospective, and randomized. Of 617 patients entered, 603 were deemed evaluable. All eligible patients had untreated, histologically confirmed D2 prostate cancer with bone or measurable soft-tissue metastases.

Both regimens were well tolerated, although a significantly increased incidence of diarrhea was noted in the combined therapy arm (13.5% vs. 5%). Analysis of variables for flare revealed that the combination reduced the flare phenomenon. There

NATIONAL CANCER INSTITUTE INTERGROUP PROTOCOL 0036
PROGRESSION-FREE SURVIVAL
CLASSIFIED BY RANDOMIZED TREATMENT
June, 1991

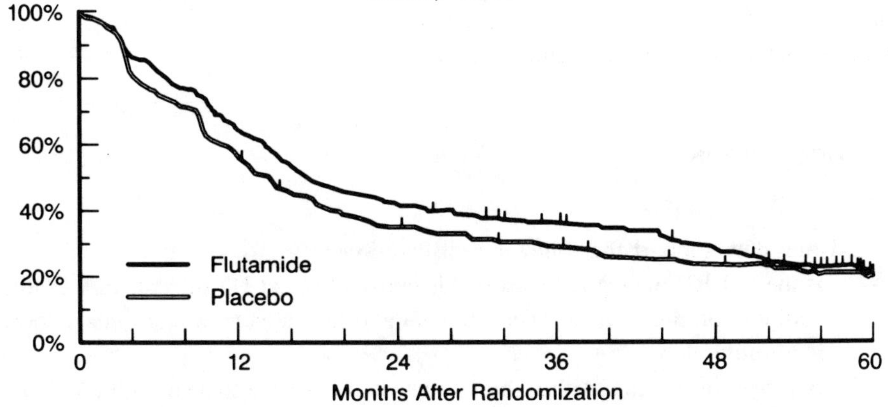

	At Risk	Events	Median in Months
Flutamide	303	242	16.9
Placebo	300	239	13.8

Figure 7-1. Androgen Therapy Study, NCI.

NATIONAL CANCER INSTITUTE INTERGROUP PROTOCOL 0036
SURVIVAL
CLASSIFIED BY RANDOMIZED TREATMENT
June, 1991

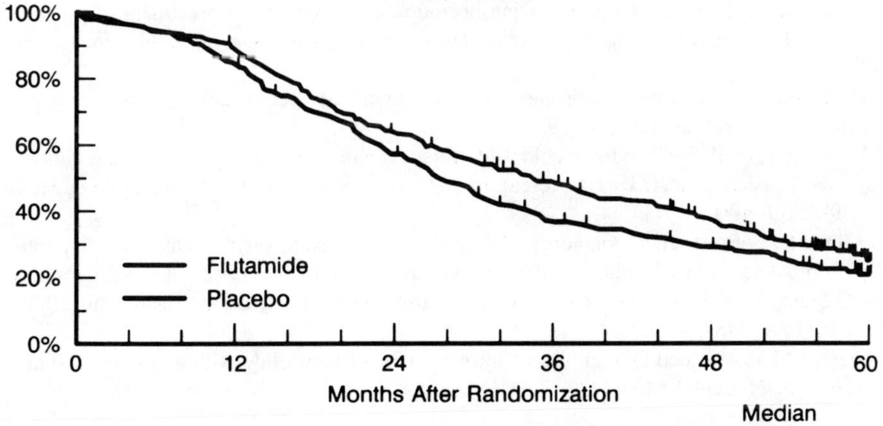

	At Risk	Deaths	Median in Months
Flutamide	303	222	35.1
Placebo	300	229	29.3

Figure 7-2. Androgen Therapy Study, (NCI).

was an increase in the time of progression from 13.8 mo to 16.9 mo (figure 7-1) and—more important—a statistically significant difference in survival rate of 35.1 mo compared to 29.3 mo with the monotherapy (figure 7-2) was noted. Most patients have benefited from this therapy; however, those with minimal disease and good performance status enjoyed even longer progression-free and overall survival rates. There is no advantage to delayed flutamide therapy.

Conclusions

Existing data support the following observations:

1. If the LH-RH analogue leuprolide is chosen to treat D2 prostate cancer, the addition of the antiandrogen flutamide offers a survival advantage over leuprolide alone.
2. A subset of patients with minimal metastatic disease treated with combination hormonal therapy appear to have a marked benefit.
3. Not all patients show a survival advantage with combined therapy, particularly those with severe disease and poor performance status.
4. The survival benefit noted in patients with minimal disease presents a research opportunity and challenge to evaluate this therapy in earlier-stage disease.

Bibliography

1. Sogani PC, Fair WR. Treatment of advanced prostatic cancer. Urol Clin North Am 1987; 14:353.
2. Crawford ED, Davis MA. Luteinizing hormone-releasing hormone analogues in the treatment of prostate cancer. In: Osborne CK, ed. Endocrine therapies in breast and prostate cancer. Boston: Kluwer Academic Publishers, 1988; 25-52.
3. Luthy I, Labrie F. Development of androgen resistance in mouse mammary tumor cells can be prevented by the antiandrogen flutamide. Prostate 1987; 10:89.
4. Beland G, Elhilali M, Fradet Y, et al. Total androgen blockade versus orchiectomy in stage D2 prostate cancer. In: Murphy GP et al, eds. Prostate cancer, Part A: research, endocrine treatment, and histopathology. New York: Alan R. Liss, 1987; 391-400.
5. Brisset JM, Boccon-Gibod L, Botto H, et al. Anandron (RV 23908) associated to surgical castration in previously untreated stage D prostate cancer: a multi-center comparative study of two doses of the drug and a placebo. In: Murphy G P et al, eds. Prostate cancer, Part A: research, endocrine treatment, and histopathology. New York: Alan R. Liss, 1987; 411-22.
6. Crawford ED, Eisenberger MA, McLeod DG, et al. A controlled trial of leuprolide with and without flutamide in prostatic carcinoma. N Engl J Med 1989; 321:419.

8

IMPACT OF CHEMOTHERAPY IN HORMONE-INDEPENDENT PROSTATE CANCER

Martin S. Tallman, M.D.

ADENOCARCINOMA OF THE PROSTATE is the second most common malignancy in American men, representing an estimated 20% of all malignant tumors in 1990. It is the third most frequent cause of cancer mortality, with a predicted 106,000 newly diagnosed cases and 30,000 deaths in 1990.[1] Early stages of the disease (stages A and B) can be cured with local therapy, either surgery or radiation, and the 5- and 10-yr survival results are 87-89% and 60-61%, respectively.[2,6]

Stage C tumors have a high rate of nodal metastases and for technical reasons are not suitable for radical surgery. Nevertheless, local control can be achieved in 80-90% of cases, and approximately 30% of patients will have a 10-yr disease-free survival time.[7-9] At time of diagnosis, however, approximately 40 percent of patients have metastatic disease (stage D), and the majority of such patients ultimately die of their disease within 4-5 yrs.[10]

Hormonal therapy with orchiectomy or estrogen administration is at present the most effective treatment for patients with stage D disease, and it provides improvement in symptoms in 70-80% of patients initially so treated. Regardless of the type of hormonal therapy chosen, the median survival duration measured from discovery of the distant metastases to death is 1-3 yr.[15] Among patients refractory to hormonal therapy, duration of survival after progression of the disease is much shorter than that of all patients with stage D disease taken as a whole. The median survival time for patients resistant to hormonal manipulation is <6 mo.[16]

Role of Nonhormonal Chemotherapy Unclear

The role of nonhormonal cytotoxic chemotherapy for hormone-refractory patients has not been clearly established. Chemotherapy studies have been difficult to conduct for several reasons. Advanced carcinoma of the prostate is manifested most frequently by positive bone scans reflecting osseous metastases that may not normalize despite improvement in symptoms. In addition, the high initial rate of response to hormonal manipulation has often limited chemotherapy studies to patients with extensive tumor burden and poor performance status. Criteria for response have included not only reduction in size of bidimensionally measurable soft-tissue tumors, but also ancillary factors, such as improvement in pain, reduction in alkaline phosphatase, and improvement in performance status, which have complicated evaluation of response. Despite these limitations, a number of studies testing various chemotherapeutic agents alone and in combinations have been carried out.

Several single agents have shown activity. At doses of >45 mg/m^2 q.3 wk, Adriamycin (ADR) has produced responses in 29% of patients.[17] Torti and colleagues at Stanford tested weekly low-dose ADR (20 mg/m^2) in 25 hormone-refractory patients and found that 4/12 patients with bidimensionally measurable tumors responded (complete remission plus partial remission [CR + PR], 33%).[18] When the National Prostate Cancer Project (NPCP) criteria for response were adhered to, the overall rate of response was 84% (CR, PR, or stable disease in 21/25 patients). Median time to failure and median survival duration from initiation of treatment were 23 wk and 41 wk, respectively. Eagan and coinvestigators reported that 5/19 patients (26%) responded to ADR 60 mg I.V. q.3 wk for 2 cycles, then q.4 wk.[24] Criteria for response in patients with both measurable and skeletal metastases only included both actual tumor measurement and assessment of ancillary factors, including pain, weight, hemoglobin, performance status, alkaline phosphatase, and acid phosphatase.

In another phase 2 study of ADR, Scher et al, using more rigid response criteria (>50% reduction in summed products of 2 diameters of all soft-tissue lesions measurable by physical examination and CT scan, lasting for >1 mo; >50% decrease in malignant hepatomegaly measured by physical examination and in all associated biochemical abnormalities and filling defects on liver scan, lasting for >1 mo; and >50% decrease of abnormally elevated serum acid phosphatase and carcinoembryonic antigen levels), found that only 2/39 patients (5%) experienced PR for (6 and 12 mo, while 3 patients had minor responses for 3-5 mo (25-49% decrease in tumor size or biochemical abnormalities lasting for >1 month or >50% decrease lasting for <1 mo) and 1 patient had stabilization of disease (<25% change in tumor size or in biochemical abnormalities over >3 mo).

Other active single agents include cisplatinum (DDP), cyclophosphamide (CTX), and 5-fluorouracil (5-FU), with objective response rates, most often using NPCP criteria, of 29-46%. The criteria, however, often included stable disease and subjective responses.[21] ADR has been shown to produce a higher response rate than a combination of 5-FU and CTX.[19] When ADR and CTX were combined in a trial involving 22 patients, objective PR was documented in 7 patients (32%), and an additional 4 patients (18%) had stable disease.[22] In this study, for patients with an objective response or stable disease, there was a significant prolongation of life compared to that of patients with progressive disease. Numerous other studies testing various combinations of the most active single agents have been conducted, with widely variable objective response rates ranging from 7 to 75%.[21]

Variable Criteria Produce Mixed Results

Variable criteria for tumor responses and frequent lack of measurable disease undoubtedly contribute to the variability of the results. Although response rates are overall somewhat higher, there is no convincing evidence that any combination is superior to single agents in controlled studies. Currently, ADR, administrated q.3 wk or in low doses on a weekly basis, has been reported to produce response rates of 15-33%, which are among the best reported for single-agent chemotherapy.[19,20,23,24] However, response has usually been defined to include minor responses and stabilization of disease. Unfortunately, many patients in this population have cardiac disease precluding the use of ADR. Most important, as yet no chemotherapeutic approach, either single-agent or combination, has demonstrated a meaningful impact on survival when tested on hormone-refractory patients.[25] Clearly, new approaches need to be explored.

5-FU is one of the single agents most thorougly studied in this setting. It has been shown to inhibit deoxyribonucleic acid synthesis and 5-alpha reductase activity in the prostatic cell.[26] The NPCP randomized patients to CTX, 5-FU, and noncytotoxic therapy (prednisone, radiation, or chlorotrianisene), and concluded that chemotherapy with either cytotoxic agent was superior to noncytotoxic therapy with respect to various measures of response. Seven of 110 evaluable patients exhibited PRs, and all responding patients were in the chemotherapy groups. A chemotherapeutic advantage was also seen in the disease category "stabilization." The number of patients who had progressive disease despite therapy was lower in the chemotherapy group than in the noncytotoxic group. In addition to more frequent objective responses, pain relief was also better in the chemotherapy group (60% vs. 26%). Although patients either responding to chemotherapy or achieving "stabilization" in the noncytotoxic group survived longer than nonresponders (60-80 wk vs. 40 wk), treatment superiority for one approach was not demonstrated.[27-30] In these studies, 5-FU was administered I.V. on a weekly basis. 5-FU is a cell cycle-specific agent, and continuous intravenous infusion may maximize its therapeutic efficacy.[31-33] Therefore, the schedule of drug administration in these studies may not have been optimal.

The difficulty in evaluating response to treatment in patients with metastatic prostate cancer is well recognized, as described above.[21, 30] A large majority of patients with metastatic disease have osseous metastases without measurable or evaluable soft-tissue or visceral disease.[34] A number of investigators have suggested alternative criteria for evaluating response to treatment,[35-37] since conventional response criteria used in other diseases are not as applicable to patients with prostate cancer.[38] Alternative response criteria have included changes in serial measurements of the serum prostatic acid phosphatase, and changes in the patient's subjective symptoms, especially bone pain. Although some investigators believe in the validity of the stable disease category,[39] others rely only on measurable or evaluable nonosseous disease for determining response in phase 2 and 3 studies.[40]

Serum acid phosphatase is a valuable biologic marker in prostate cancer, and its measurement has become important in staging and in following response to treatment. However, it has limitations, including its frequent lack of elevation in early disease and a potential lack of elevation in patients with undifferentiated tumors, making it useless as a screening test. The NPCP concluded that a 50% reduction in tumor mass, relief of pain, and a decrease in the acid phosphatase after chemotherapy were positively correlated.[41] This was confirmed in another study. However, in 10% of cases, progression of disease was noted despite declining levels of acid phosphatase.[42]

Use of PSA Marker in Evaluating Patients

Prostate-specific antigen (PSA) is a new biochemical marker useful in the evaluation of patients with prostate cancer.[43-44] PSA is a glycoprotein found only in the ductal epithelium of prostate tissue, normal or malignant. The level of this marker is elevated in >90% of patients with metastatic prostate cancer,[5] and may be a useful predictor of response to treatment of patients with prostate cancer.[46] A prognostic relationship between pretreatment levels of PSA and patient survival among those with advanced disease has been suggested.[47] Pointes et al, using serial PSA levels in patients with stages B2 to D disease, found an excellent correlation between elevated levels and the development of metastatic disease in a group undergoing prostatectomy.[48] Following radical prostatectomy, the level of PSA reliably falls to undetectable levels, and monitoring the PSA level may be useful in detecting residual disease or early recurrence following surgery and in evaluating response to radiotherapy.[49] However, the impact of chemotherapy on the level of PSA and its value in evaluating and predicting response to chemotherapy among patients with hormone-resistant disease has not been thoroughly studied.

At the Northwestern University Cancer Center, we have begun a study evaluating the impact of continuous infusion 5-FU in the treatment of advanced (stage D3) adenocarcinoma of the prostate. Thirteen patients have been treated with monthly 5-FU (1,000 mg/m^2) for $\leq$5 mo. Patients have been evaluated clinically and with serial prostate-specific antigen (PSA) levels, prostatic acid phosphatase (PAP) levels, and bone scans. Seven patients have had no response by objective measured parameters. Five patients have had stabilization (<25% decline in PSA or plateau of previously rising levels) of disease. One patient had a clinical PR (> 50% decline in PSA and improved bone scan); however, he received simultaneous pelvic irradiation. Drug toxicity included mucositis in 7 patients, 4 requiring dose modifications. The study thus far shows that continuous infusion 5-FU is feasible and may have clinical efficacy in patients with advanced prostate cancer, warranting further clinical trials in better performance level patients and earlier in the natural history of their disease.

Conclusion

In conclusion, active agents against prostate cancer include ADR, 5-FU, DDP, and CTX. Combination chemotherapy has not proven superior to single agents. Pain relief and palliation can be achieved with chemotherapy. Chemotherapy has not been shown definitively to improve survival. New agents with activity need to be explored with patients entered onto clinical trials. One needs to use rigidly defined objective measurements for tumor response. New markers of disease activity, such as the PSA, may afford the opportunity to better explore the efficacy of newly identified active agents as well as older active agents perhaps not optimally used in the past.

References

1. American Cancer Society: 1990 Cancer Facts and Figures. New York: American Cancer Society, 1990.
2. Boxer RJ. Adenocarcinoma of the prostate gland. Urol Serv 1977; 27:75.
3. Jewett HJ. The present status of radical prostatectomy for Stage A and B prostate cancer. Urol Clin North Am 1975; 2:105.
4. Correa RJ Jr, Gibbons RP, Cummings KB, Mason JT. Total prostatectomy for Stage B carcinoma of the prostate. J Urol 1975; 117:328.
5. Hodges CV, Pearse HD, Stille I. Radical prostatectomy for carcinoma: 30-year experience and 15-year survivals. J Urol 1979; 122:180.
6. Walsh PC, Jewett HJ. Radical surgery for prostate cancer. Cancer 1980; 45: 1906.
7. Perez CA, Baur W, Garza R, Rouce RK. Radiation therapy in the definitive treatment of localized carcinoma of the prostate. Cancer 1977; 40:1425.
8. McGowen DG. Radiation therapy in the management of localized carcinoma of the prostate: a preliminary report. Cancer 1977; 39:98-103.
9. Bagshaw MA. Radiation therapy for cancer of the prostate. In: Skinner DG, de Kernion JB, eds. Genitourinary cancer. Philadelphia: WB Saunders Co, 1978; 355-379.
10. Mellinger GT, Bailar JD III, Arduino LJ, et al. Treatment and survival of patients with cancer of the prostate. Surg Gynecol Obstet 1967; 4:1011-17.
11. Mobley, TL, Frank IN. Influence of tumor grade or survival and on serum acid phosphatase levels in metastatic carcinoma of the prostate. J Urol 1968; 99:321.
12. Resnick MI, Grayhack JT. Treatment of Stage IV carcinoma of the prostate. Urol Clin North Am 1978; 2:141-161.

13. Nesbit RM, Plumb RT. Prostatic carcinoma: a follow-up on 795 patients treated prior to the endocrine era and a comparison of survival rates between these and patients treated by endocrine therapy. Surgery 1946; 20:263-72.
14. Blackard CE, Byar DP, Jordan WP Jr, et al. Orchiectomy for advanced prostatic carcinoma: a re-evaluation. Urology 1973; 1:553-60.
15. Bailor JL, Byar DP. Estrogen treatment for cancer of the prostate. Cancer 1970; 26:257-61.
16. Johnson DE, Scott WW, Gibbons RP, et al. National randomized study of chemotherapeutic agents in advanced prostatic carcinoma: a progress report. Cancer Treat Rep 1977; 61:317-23.
17. O'Bryan RM, Baker LH, Gottlieb JE, et al. Dose response evaluation of Adriamycin in human neoplasia. Cancer 1977; 39:1940-48.
18. Torti FM, Aston D, Lum BL, et al. Weekly doxorubicin in endocrine-refractory carcinoma of the prostate. J Clin Oncol 1983; 1:477-82.
19. Egan RT, Hahn RG, Myers RP. Adriamycin versus 5-Fluorouracil and cyclophosphamide in the treatment of metastatic cancer. Cancer Treat Rep 1976; 60:115-17.
20. Scher H, Yagoda A, Watson RC, Serber M, Whitmore, W. Phase II trial of doxorubicin in bidimensionally measurable prostatic adenocarcinoma. J Urol 1984; 131:1099-1102.
21. Torti FM, Carter SK. The chemotherapy of prostatic adenocarcinoma. Ann Intern Med 1980; 92:681-89.
22. Ihde DC, Bonn PA, Cohen MH, Donnick NR, Eddy JL, Minna JD. Effective treatment of hormonally-unresponsive metastatic carcinoma of the prostate with Adriamycin and cyclophosphamide. Cancer 1980; 45:1300-10.
23. O'Bryan RM, Baker LH, Gottlieb JF, et al. Dose responsive evaluation of Adriamycin in human neoplasia. Cancer 1977; 39:1940-48.
24. Torti, Aston D. Lum BL, et al. Weekly doxorubicin in endocrine refractory carcinoma of the prostate. J Clin Oncol 1983; 1:477-82.
25. Eisenberger MA, Simon R, O'Dwyer PJ, Wittes RE, Friedman MA. A re-evaluation of non-hormonal cytotoxic chemotherapy in the treatment of prostatic carcinoma. J Clin Oncol 1985; 3:827-40.
26. Saroff J, Kirdani R, Yamanka H, Murphy GP, Sandberg AA. A possible model for drugs in prostatic carcinoma. Proc Am Assoc Cancer Res 1973; 14:13.
27. Scott W, Johnson DE, Schmidt, JE, et al. Chemotherapy of advanced prostatic cancer with cyclophosphamide or 5-fluorouracil: results of first national randomized study. J Urol 1976; 114: 909-11.
28. Scott WW, Gibbons, RP, Johnson DE, et al. Comparison of 5-fluorouracil (NSC-019893) and cyclophosphamide (SC-026271) in patients with advanced carcinoma of the prostate. Cancer Chemother Res 1975; 59:105-201.
29. Scott WW, Gibbons RP, Johnson DE, et al. The continued evaluation of the effects of chemotherapy in patients with advanced carcinoma of the prostate. J Urol 1976; 116:211-13.
30. Schmidt JD, Johnson DE, Scot WW, Gibbons RP, Prout GR, Murphy GP. Chemotherapy of advanced prostatic cancer: evaluation of response paramters. Urology 1976; 121:185-89.
31. Siefert P, Baker LH, Reed ML, Vaitkevicius VK. Comparison of continuously infused 5-fluorouracil with bolus injection in treatment of patients with colorectal adenocarcinoma. Cancer 1975; 36:123-28.
32. Hum GJ, Bateman JR. 5 day IV infusion with 5-fluorouracil (5-FU; NSC-19893) for gastroenteric carcinoma after failure on weekly 5-FU therapy. Cancer Chemother Rep. Pt I 1975; 59(6):1177-79.
33. Moertel CG, Schutt AJ, Reiteman RJ, et al. A comparison of fluorouracil administered by slow infusion and rapid injection. Cancer Res 1972; 32:2717-19.
34. Hovesepian JA, Byar DP, Veterans Administration Cooperative Urological Research Group. Carcinoma of the prostate: correlation between radiographic quantitation of metastases and patient survival. Urology 1975; 6:11-15.
35. Ihde DC, Bunn PA, Cohen MH, Dunnick NR, Eddy HL, Minna JD. Effective treatment of hormonally-unresponsive metastatic carcinoma of the prostate with Adriamycin and cyclophosphamide: methods of documenting tumor response and progression. Cancer 1980; 45:1300-10.

36. Davlson DF, Berry WR, Cox EB, Walker A, Lazlo J. Treatment of metastatic endocrine-unresponsive carcinoma of the prostate gland with multi-agent chemotherapy: indicators of response to treatment. JNCI 1979; 63:615-22.
37. Kvols LK, Egan RT, Myers RP. Evaluation of melphalan, ICRF-159, and hydroxyurea in metastatic prostate cancer: a preliminary report. Cancer Treat Rep 1979; 61:311-12.
38. Haywood SL, Carbone PR, Hevson JC, Kumaoka S, Segaloff A, Rubens RD. Assessment of response to therapy in advanced breast cancer. Cancer 1977; 39:1289-94.
39. Slack NH, Mittelman A, Brady MF, Murphy GP. The importance of the stable category for chemotherapy treated patients with advanced and relapsing prostate cancer. Cancer 1980; 46:2393-2402.
40. Yagoda A, Watson RC, Natale RB, et al. A critical analysis of response criteria in patients with prostate cancer treated with cisdiammine dichloride platinum II. Cancer 1979; 44:1553-62.
41. Johnson DE, Prout GR, Scott WW, et al. Clinical significance of serum acid phosphatase levels in advanced prostatic carcinoma. Urology 1976; 8:123-126.
42. Richards B, Sylvester R, dePaun M, et al. The clinical value of the serum acid phosphatase in carcinoma of the prostate. In: Pavone-Macaluso M, Smith PH, eds. Cancer of the prostate and kidney. New York: Dlonum, 1981; 167-77.
43. Nadji M. Tabei SZ, Castro A, et al. Prostatic-specific antigen: an immunohistologic marker for prostatic neoplasms. Cancer 1981; 48:1229-32.
44. Killian CS, Yang N, Emrich LJ, et al, and the investigators of the National Prostate Cancer Project. Cancer Res 1985; 45:886-91.
45. Kuriyama M, Wange MC, Lee CL, et al. Multiple marker evaluation in human prostate cancer with the use of tissue-specific antigens. JNCI 1982; 68:99-105.
46. Kuriyama M, Wang MC, Papsidero LD, et al. Quantitation of prostate-specific antigen in monitoring prostate cancer. Cancer Res 1981; 41:3874-76.
47. Kuriyama M, Wang MC, Lee CL, et al. The use of human prostate-specific antigen in monitoring prostate cancer. Cancer Res 1981; 41:3874-76.
48. Pointes JE, Chu TM, Slack NH, Karr J, Murphy GP. Serum prostate antigen measurement in localized prostate cancer: correlation with clinical course. J Urol 1982; 128:1216-20.

9

SALVAGE RADICAL PROSTATECTOMY FOR RADIORECURRENT ADENOCARCINOMA OF THE PROSTATE

Robert P. Weaver, M.D., and
Peter T. Scardino, M.D.

RADIOTHERAPY IS A WIDELY used treatment modality in early-stage prostate cancer. Although long-term survival rates have been satisfactory, local tumor recurrence or persistence has been reported with distressing frequency in patients treated with definitive radiotherapy (XRT).[1] Patients who have a positive biopsy after XRT have a much greater chance of local recurrence and distant metastases than do patients with a negative biopsy result.[2] We have investigated the role of salvage radical prostatectomy for selected patients with local recurrence after XRT.[3]

Criteria for Study of 30 Patients

Patients with biopsy-proven tumor 12 mo or more after definitive XRT were considered potential candidates for salvage prostatectomy. The indications for biopsy included a persistent or enlarging palpable nodule in 22 patients, and abnormal ultrasound or rising prostate-specific antigen (PSA) level in 4 patients, an incidentally discovered cancer at transurethral resection of the prostate for bladder outlet obstruction in 3 patients, and a routine positive postirradiation biopsy result in 1 patient. All patients had an early stage tumor (stage A2, B or small C) and negative pelvic lymph nodes (if a lymph node dissection was performed) at time of initial treatment. All patients were in excellent general health with a life expectancy of at least 10 yr. They had received no previous hormonal therapy that might mask occult metastases.

Physical examination, transrectal ultrasongraphy, PSA (when available), prostatic acid phosphatase, and bone scan results were consistent with localized disease.

All patients then underwent urodynamic investigations, cystoscopy, examination under anesthesia, proctoscopy, and evaluation of the upper urinary tract. The clinical stage and grade of the tumor at the time of recurrence are summarized in table 9-1. This was a heavily pretreated group of patients: 23 patients had had a pelvic lymphadenectomy, and 21 patients had radioactive seed implantation. Only 7 patients had been treated with external beam therapy alone with no previous pelvic surgery. All patients were fully informed of the increased risks associated with a salvage operation, including urinary incontinence, impotence, and rectal injury.

Table 9-1. Clinical Stage and Grade of Tumor at Recurrence in 30 Patients

Stage	N(%)
A2	8* (27)
B1	15 (50)
B2	7 (23)
Total	30 (100)
Grade	**N(%)**
I	1 (3)
II	20 (67)
III	5 (17)
Unknown	4 (13)
Total	30 (100)

*Patients had no nodule at time of recurrence. Biopsy performed by needle in 5 cases and TUR in 3 cases.

All patients underwent an antibiotic and mechanical bowel preparation because of the risk of injury to the rectum. The procedure was initiated through a perineal incision so that the rectum could be separated from the prostate under direct vision and the maximum posterior periprostatic tissue could be removed. The urethra was transected distal to the apex and the perineal wound closed. The patient was then placed supine, and a retropubic approach was used to mobilize the adherent bladder and prostate. The dissection was performed in a retrograde fashion, made easier by the plane of dissection already achieved between prostate and rectum. The bladder neck was divided from the prostate and the specimen removed. The bladder neck was then reconstructed with mucosal eversion, and the vesicourethral anastomosis was performed in the standard fashion.

Results

Among the first 30 patients at our institution, there have been no operative deaths. The operation averaged 4.5 hr, compared to 3.0 hr for a standard pelvic lymphadenectomy and radical retropubic prostatectomy. The average hospital stay was somewhat longer (9.8 days) than for a standard radical prostatectomy, but the blood loss was less. Complications, particularly those related to an operation in an irradiated field, are listed in table 9-2. Fifteen patients suffered no complications. Among 24 patients followed for >1 yr, 13 (54%) became continent (no more than 1 pad per day) at an average of 4½ mo after the operation. Eleven patients (46%) remained incontinent (2 or more pads per day) and 6 of these are dry after placement of an artificial urinary sphincter.

Table 9-2. Complications

Type	N (%)
Rectal Injury	6 (20)
Closed without complications	4
Rectal injury leading to further surgery (colostomy, vesicorectal fistula repair)	2
Anastomotic stricture*	7 (23)
Ureteral transection	1 (3)
Ureterovesical junction stricture	1 (3)

*1 patient developed 2 strictures.

To assess the extent of the disease accurately, the pathologist inked the entire specimen to document the margins of resection. Transverse whole-mount step sections were examined histologically. Table 9-3 summarizes the pathologic findings. Tumor was confined to the prostate or periprostatic tissue with negative seminal vesicles and negative surgical margins in 12 patients (40%).

These patients have been followed postoperatively for a mean of 32 mo (range: 2-70 mo). Interval assessment has included physical examination, determination of serum acid phosphatase and PSA levels, and bone scan when indicated. The current status of the patients is summarized in Table 9-4. At this writing, 16 patients are alive with no evidence of recurrent cancer; 14 of these have a serum PSA level <0.4 ng/ml (Hybritech), while the PSA level in 2 patients is not yet available. Eleven patients have evidence of recurrence, including all patients with a PSA level >0.4 ng/ml. Twenty-seven patients are alive and 3 patients are dead. Only 1 patient has died of prostate cancer; the other 2 died without evidence of recurrent disease.

Table 9-3. Summary of Pathologic Findings in 30 Patients

Findings	N(%)
Confined to prostate or perioprostatic tissue; seminal vesicles and surgical margins negative	12 (40)
Microscopic seminal vesicle invasion (negative margins)	8 (27)
Positive margins (includes 7 who also had seminal vesicle invasion)	8 (27)
Positive nodes	2 (6)
Total	30 (100)

Table 9-4. Current Status of 30 Patients (Mean Follow-up 32 Mo; Range 2-70 Mo)

	N (%)	N (%)
Alive	27 (90)	
No recurrence (PSA $\leq$0.4)		16 (53)
Recurrence (PSA $\leq$0.4, positive bone scan, positive nodes)		11 (11)
Dead	3 (10)	
Never recurred		2 (71)
2° to prostate cancer		1 (3)
Total	30 (100)	

Preoperative PSA levels and transrectal ultrasonography were found to reflect accurately the pathological extent of the disease. Postoperative PSA levels have correlated well with the extent of tumor in the specimen, but PSA levels have remained normal thus far in some patients with seminal vesicle invasion and positive surgical margins.

Our series included a highly select group of healthy individuals with well-documented local recurrence of prostate cancer after XRT in whom options for cure were limited. We believe that salvage prostatectomy is a technically feasible procedure with acceptable morbidity and provides excellent local control in such patients. At least in the intermediate term ($\pm$5 yr), eradication of cancer can be achieved in a reasonable proportion of patients.

References

1. Scardino PT, Wheeler TM. Local control of prostate cancer with radiotherapy: frequency and prognostic significance of positive results of postirradiation prostate biopsy. NCI Monogr 1988; 7:95.
2. Scardino PT, Frankel JM, Wheeler TM, et al. The prognostic significance of postirradiation biopsy results in patients with prostatic cancer. J Urol 1986; 135:510.
3. Meacham RB, Scardino PT. Salvage radical prostatectomy for recurrent prostate cancer after radiotherapy. World J Urol 1989; 7:51.

10

GROWTH FACTOR INHIBITORS IN HORMONE REFRACTORY PROSTATIC CANCER: THE ROLE OF SURAMIN

Howard I. Scher, M.D.; Jacqueline M. Iversen, R.Ph.; Tracy Curley, R.N.; and William Tong, Ph.D.

Introduction

IN THE SEARCH FOR novel anticancer treatments, it is easy to neglect compounds that are already available. Suramin, the hexasodium salt of 8,8'-[carbonylbis[imino-3,1-phenylenecarbonylimino (4-methyl-3,1-phenylene)carbonylimino]] bis-1,3,5-naphthalenesulfonic acid (figure 10-1), is one such example. Interest in the compound, which was originally synthesized in 1916 and used to used to treat trypanosomiasis and onchocerciasis in the 1920s,[1,2] waned until 1979, when suramin was found to reduce viremia in patients with AIDS and to inhibit reverse transcriptase.[3,4] Subsequently, suramin was shown to inhibit growth factor binding and growth factor-induced mitogenesis in vitro at concentrations achievable in the clinic.[5] This led to clinical trials in both hematologic malignancies and solid tumors. Prostate cancer, in particular, was targeted for evaluation due to suramin's inhibition of growth factor action, its effects on human prostate derived cell lines in vitro, and its known adrenal inhibitory effects.[6]

Mechanisms

The ability of suramin to inhibit growth factor binding in vitro correlates well with its ability to inhibit cell growth as measured by inhibition of DNA systhesis,

Supported by National Cancer Institute CA-05826, CM-55732.

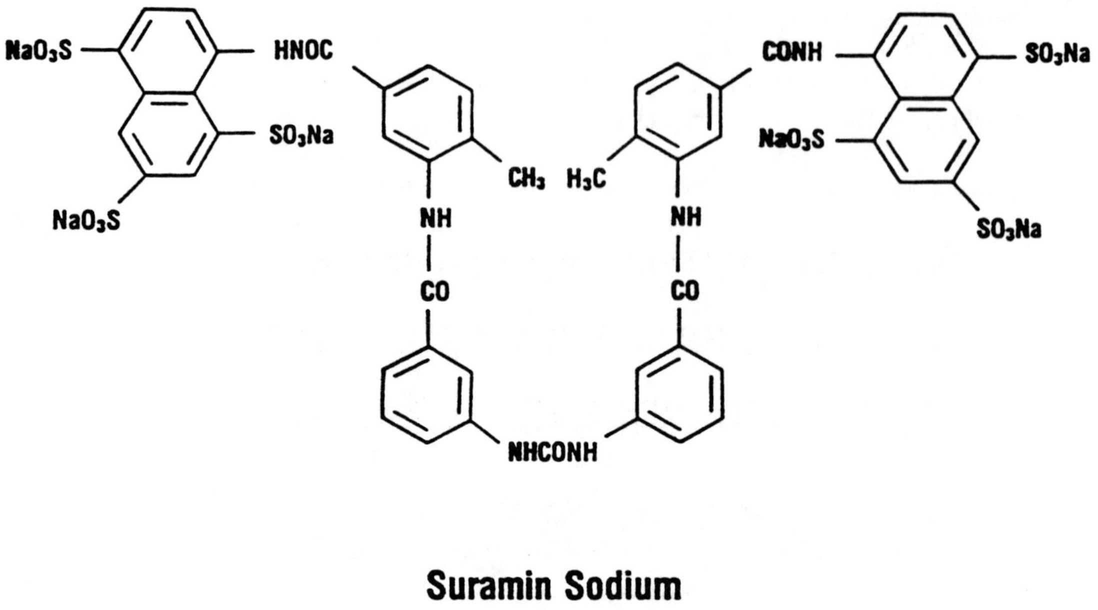

Figure 1. The structure of sodium suramin.

by assays of cell number, and by its effects on colony-forming ability. The effects vary with (1) the concentration of suramin, (2) duration of suramin exposure, (3) concentration of serum in the medium, and (4) the number and type of cells plated. For example, a suramin concentration that had minimal effect on epidermal growth factor (EGF) induced mitogenesis of AKR-2B cells[7] and blocked EGF mitogenesis on LNCaP cells by >90%.[8] The drug is extensively protein bound, and its action can be inhibited by albumin.[9] Other growth factors inhibited in vitro include basic and acidic fibroblast growth factors (FGF) and transforming growth factors (TGF) α and β.[10-12]

The actions of suramin are not restricted to growth factor inhibition. Other actions include inhibition of lysosomal enzymes, including hyaluronidase, iduronate sulfatase, β-glucuronidase, and sphingoid hydrolases.[13,14] The effect on lysosomal enzyme synthesis results in a systemic accumulation of glycosoaminoglycans (GAGs) and sphingolipids mimicking the pathology associated with mucopolysaccharidosis.[15] GAGs, primarily heparan and dermatan sulfate, accumulate in the serum, urine, kidney, liver, lung, and spleen.[13] This explains some of the unique toxicities of the compound. Suramin also inhibits nucleic acid polymerases,[16] membrane-associated ion pumps such as NaK, Ca and H+−ATPases,[17] protein kinase C,[18] and glycolysis,[19] and induces differentiation of HT29 colon carcinoma cell lines.[20]

Growth Factors and the Prostate

One proposed mechanism of androgen escape is autocrine production of growth factors that previously required androgen stimulation for production. A number of growth factors have been identified from conditioned media of human-derived prostate cancer cell lines and from rat and human prostate tissues, both benign and malignant. These include basic and acidic FGF, TGF α, TGF β, insulin-like growth factor-1 (ILGF-1), EGF, platelet-derived growth factor (PDGF), and other unclassified mitogens.[11,12,21-31] Although the actions and interactions of these factors are complex and the relative contribution of each factor – alone or in combination – is unknown, fibroblast growth factors seem to be present in the highest relative proportion. Using a variety of cellular targets (3T3 fibroblasts, MC3T3-El osteoblasts, endothelial cells, and prostate epithelial cells [benign and malignant, rat and human]), FGFs have been implicated in the angiogenesis, stromal growth, osteoblastic growth, and malignant prostatic epithelial cell growth in vivo.[21,24-30]

In addition, evidence exists for a functional TGF α and EGF autocrine loop in prostate cancer cell growth and proliferation. This has been shown by the observations that (1) the growth factor is synthesized by prostate cancer cells,[22,23] (2) the specific receptor, the epidermal growth factor receptor (EGFr), can be isolated on the cell surface;[23] (3) addition of TGF α or EGF to culture media increases cell growth and proliferation;[8,21-23] and (4) specific antibodies that block the binding of TGF α and EGF to the receptor inhibit cell growth.[31] Independent studies have shown that transfection of a TGF α gene under the influence of a viral promoter in the mouse prostate reconstitution system produces hypertrophic growth of the prostate.[32] Suramin can inhibit this loop.[33]

Cell Line Studies In Vitro

Suramin has been shown to produce growth inhibition by at least 50% of the PC-3,[34,35] DU-145,[34] and by >97% using LNCaP human-derived prostate cancer cell lines at a concentration of 100 μM (150 μg/ml).[35] With DU-145 cells, growth-inhibitory effects were partially reversed by exogenous androgens or EGF/TGF α,[8] and in LNCaP cells by bFGF,[30,34] EGF, and testosterone.[34] Greater inhibition of PC-3 cell growth was seen with increased concentrations and/or longer durations of exposure. As shown in table 10-1, if cells are rinsed free of suramin after 5 days, cell growth continues. This implies a cytostatic as opposed to cytocidal effect. However, if suramin (100 μM) is maintained for 10 days, an 87% inhibition of growth is observed, suggesting a cytocidal effect.[36] The relative effect of different serum concentrations was shown by comparing the IC_{50} in 2 versus 10% serum. An increase from 30 to 300 μM was noted.[34] In this system, cytotoxicity was observed after 3 days' exposure, with evidence of mitochondrial damage on histological examination.[37]

Table 10-1. Effect of Prolonged Exposure to Suramin on PC-3 Cells

Treatment		Cell # ($\times10^4$)
Plated	day 0	1.0
Control	day 6	16.6±1.0
Suramin	day 6	9.4±1.0
Rinsed	day 12	56.2±2.3
Suramin	day 12	1.2±0.1

Ten thousand PC-3 cells were plated and the following day 100 μM suramin was added; 5 days later (6 days after plating) the cells were counted or rinsed, fresh media added, and the incubation continued with or without the presence of 100 μM suramin.
Source: ref 36

The effects also have been examined in human prostate primary epithelial cultures. Again, an effect on growth factor-induced mitogenesis was reversible up to 6 days. Thereafter, cytotoxicity was observed. Of potentially greater importance was the observed differential effects at various serum concentrations. Levels above $10^{-4}M$ were inhibitory, while stimulation was observed in a range of 5 X 10^{-7} to $10^{-5}M$ in 9 out of 14 cultures.[38] A similar outcome was observed in the Dunning rat tumor model. Although suramin inhibited growth of the R3327-AT-2 variant,[12] it stimulated growth of the R3327-AT-3 and MAT-LYLU variants.[35] The differential inhibition may reflect suramin's blockade of growth factors known to inhibit cell growth such as TGF β and may have important clinical implications.[39]

Clinical Trials

Pharmacologic Studies

The first trials investigated a weekly I.V. dose schedule. Toxicities were prohibitive, leading to studies using continuous infusion (C.I.). According to these dosing guidelines, a 200-mg test dose is administered, followed by a C.I. of 350 mg/m^2/day. Because suramin inhibits adrenal enzyme synthesis, all patients are given hydrocortisone replacement from the initiation of treatment. Therapy is continued until the target concentration of 280-300 μg/ml, the upper limit of the "therapeutic window." Beyond this, the frequency of dose-limiting toxicities increases dramatically. The lower limit was based on phase 1 investigations, where no responses were observed in 4 patients who did not achieve levels of >200 μg/ml. Dose-limiting toxicities increase dramatically above 300 μg/ml.[40-42] A nomogram was developed for weekly dose adjustments, depending on the plasma suramin concentrations. Because of the observed half-life (t½) in previous trials, retreatment of responding patients was planned at 2- to 3-mo intervals.[42]

Based on promising results reported by the NCI, *vide infra*, a confirmatory trial was initiated using the dosing schedule previously described. In the context of this trial, additional pharmacology studies were performed. Significant interpatient variation in measured suramin concentrations was noted. In addition, the observed t½ was much shorter than previously reported (15-30 days in several cases).[43] Subsequently, a computer model was developed to individualize dosage regimens. Using published literature values and derived pharmacokinetic parameters from daily plasma concentrations during the loading phase of treatment, a maximum a posteriori Bayesian pharmacokinetic parameters value estimator was designed.[44] With this method, levels obtained on days 1 and 2 are used to predict levels on day 3, levels on days 1 and 3 used to predict day 4, etc. The model allows for the calculation of dosing regimens for both C.I. or intermittent bolus treatments.[43] An example of the measured (o) versus the model or computer predicted (+) concentrations using the NCI schedule is shown in figure 10-2. As illustrated, a second infusion was started when the trough level reached 100 μg/ml, about 22 days after achieving a target concentration of 290 μg/ml. Other groups have investigated more rapid infusions (400-600 mg/m²/day) until the target suramin concentration is achieved.[45,46] At present, the optimal dosing regimen has not been defined.

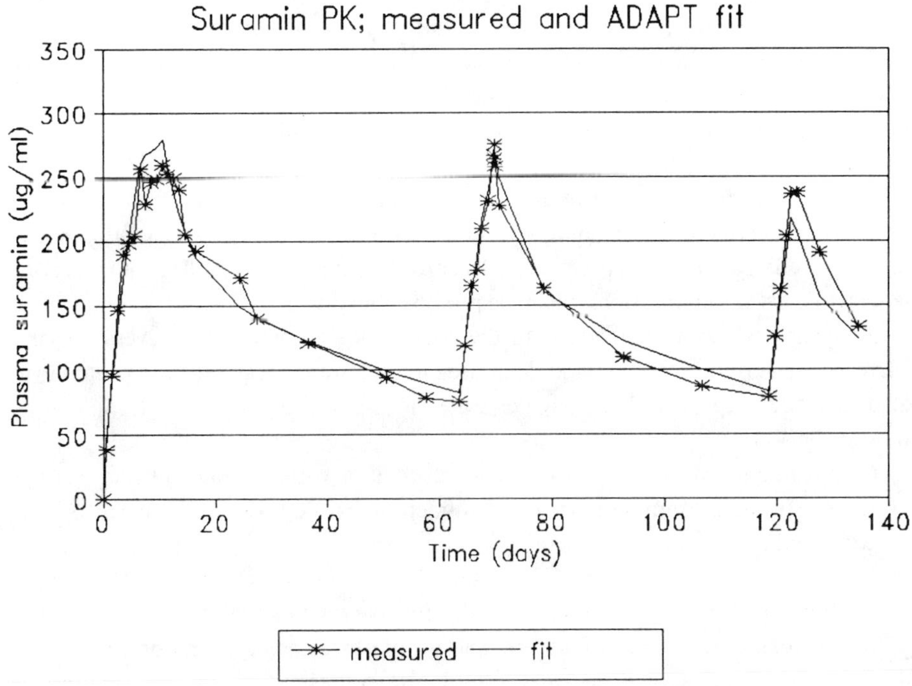

Figure 10-2. Plot of the predicted (*) and measured (+) plasma suramin concentrations using the MAP-Bayesian PK estimator[43] in a patient with measurable prostatic cancer treated at 350 mg/m²/day by continuous infusion.

Available pharmacokinetic data suggest that suramin disposition in plasma can be described by a 2-compartment model.[40,43] In the first 1-2 wk of therapy, disappearance from the plasma is best described by the distributional clearance (CL_D). As equilibrium is approached between the plasma and peripheral tissues, the disappearance is described by the total plasma clearance (CL_T). Using this schema clinically, an initial dose that loads the central compartment, followed by tapering doses to achieve a final steady state, would allow a therapeutic target to be achieved rapidly and levels to be maintained in a defined range. The presence of a third or multiple compartments is suggested by the accumulation of suramin over time unaccounted for in a 2-compartment model. This has not been fully characterized. At present, it is also unknown whether free or bound (>99%) suramin is the active moiety. This may prove difficult to characterize as a reproducible assay, because the free compound has not been developed.[47]

Toxicity Profile

Use of suramin contrasts significantly with classical chemotherapy because the agent has several unique toxicities. Many adverse effects are mediated by the inhibition of glycosaminoglycan synthesis and growth factors. Among the most worrisome is a polyradiculopathy progressing to a Guillain-Barré syndrome. An inhibitory effect on FGF, a growth factor for Schwann cells, has been postulated. Risk of toxicity correlates with peak suramin levels, exceeding 40% at >350 μg/ml.[48] It is unclear, however, whether longer durations of treatment at lower plasma concentrations will have the same effect on nerve cells.

A coagulopathy, the result of accumulation of heparan and chondroitan sulfate, which function as circulating anticoagulants, has been reported. This can be particularly severe in patients with preexisting liver dysfunction. As a result, protocols contain provisions to stop infusions when the prothrombin time is >17 sec. Discontinuance of the drug leads to normalization of the coagulation parameters in several days.[49] Increases in serum creatinine and decreases in creatinine clearance and proteinuria also have been reported. This may be related to the selective accumulation of suramin in the kidney.[50]

Glycoaminoglycan inhibition can also result in a vortex keratopathy in ≤25% of cases. Slit lamp examinations reveal intraepithelial deposits in the cornea, conjunctiva, and lens epithelia. Electron microscopy shows lipid inclusion lamellar membranous bodies similar to Fabry's disease.[51] Symptoms, which include blurring of vision, photophobia, and tearing, generally resolve when suramin is discontinued.

An increased incidence of severe and/or life-threatening infections has been documented in patients with normal granulocyte counts.[41,52,53] No consistent effect on neutrophil function has been observed.[52] Hypocalcemia, liver function abnormalities, pericardial effusion, anaphylaxis, nausea, vomiting, urticaria, fever, rash, lymphopenia, and thrombocytopenia also have been reported.[41,54]

Results in Prostatic Cancer

As previously noted, the impetus to evaluate suramin in patients with prostatic cancer was based on its antitumor activity against prostatic cancer cell lines in vitro and in vivo, its inhibitory effects on growth factor-induced mitogenesis and proliferation, and its effects on the adrenal steroidogenesis. In the first study at the National Cancer Institute (NCI) a decrease of ≥50% was observed in 7/11 (63%) cases (63%), whereas 4/8 patients showed >50% regression in measurable disease.[55] Subsequently, a confirmatory trial using the same dose schedule was started at the University of Texas M.D. Anderson Cancer Center, the Mayo Clinic, and the Memorial Sloan-Kettering Cancer Center. Of the first 17 evaluable patients, partial remission (PR) was noted in 2 (12%, 95% confidence limits 0-27%), and decreases in PSA (>50%) in 3/14 evaluable cases. Accrual will continue until 40 patients have been evaluated.[54]

The NCI later updated its experience with 35 patients—15 with measurable lesions, 21 with painful bony lesions, and 29 with a baseline PSA >5 times normal. Overall response in measurable disease was observed in 6 (40%; 3 with no change in PSA), and an improvement in bone pain was noted in 15 (70%). Evaluating only PSA, 6 (21%) had a normalization, whereas a total of 16 (55%) had at least a 50% decrease from baseline. The median survival was 9 mo for those with soft-tissue disease and 15 mo for those with disease limited to the skeleton.[56]

The results reported by other groups using a variety of dosing schedules is shown in table 10-2. Ahmann et al noted PR in measurable disease in 6/14 evaluable cases, with a >80% decrease in PSA in 6 (43%, 95 confidence limits 17-69%).[53] Using the same schedule, Dawson et al noted PSA responses in 10 (50%) of patients

Table 10-2. Reported Results Using Suramin in Prostatic Cancer

		Measurable Disease			PSA Response		
Reference	Schedule	No.	PR	(95% conf)	No.	PR	(95% conf)
56	Infusion	15	6(40%)	(15-65%)	19	29(66%)	(48-83%)
57	Infusion		NR*		20	10(50%)	(28-72%)
45	Infusion		NR		9	4(44%)	(12-77%)
58	Infusion		NR		5	3(60%)	(17-100%)
54	Infusion	17	2(12%)	(0-27%)	14	3 (21%)	(0-43%)
59	Interm	4	4(100%)		7	6(86%)	(60-100%)
53	Infusion	14	6(43%)	17-69%)	14	6(43%)	(17-69%)
67**	Infusion	25	5(20%)	(4-36%)		NR	
Total		77	23(30%)	(20-40%)	95	51(54%)	(44-64%)

*NR = not reported
** + mitomycin C

treated.[57] In 2 other studies in which a slightly different infusion schedule was used, response in PSA was observed in 3/5[58] and 4/9 cases,[45] respectively. More recently, Eisenberger et al,[58] using an intermittent schedule based on a modified a priori Bayesian pharmacokinetic parameter (MAP-PK) estimator,[43] noted regression in soft-tissue disease in 3/3 and >50% decrease in PSA in 8/9 evaluable cases.[59] In most studies, response durations are generally short.[58]

Discussion and Conclusions

The reported results show that suramin has activity in hormone-refractory prostatic cancer. Considering measurable disease sites, a 30% response proportion (95% confidence limits 20-40%) a ≥50% decrease in PSA was observed in 54% of cases (95% confidence limits 44-64%). This is higher than reported for other chemotherapeutic agents or secondary hormonal manipulations. Further investigation of suramin is warranted, but practical and reproducible dosing regimens need to be developed. In this regard, the report by Eisenberger et al is of interest; responses were observed in 8/9 cases using an intermittent schedule designed to maintain levels in a therapeutic range.[59] A parallel study at Memorial Sloan-Kettering is ongoing.

Alternatively, one could argue that suramin has modest antitumor activity. A comparison of the survival distributions of patients treated at the NCI with those of a group of 146 patients with measurable hormone refractory disease treated with chemotherapy at Memorial Sloan-Kettering showed no difference.[61] Perhaps the results are due to hydrocortisone alone. For example, ketoconazole and prednisone have been reported to decrease measurable PSA concentrations by ≥50% in 80% (12/15) of cases.[62] Hydrocortisone alone has also been shown to palliate pain and improve quality of life.[63] A randomized trial of suramin plus hydrocortisone versus hydrocortisone alone was initiated to address this question, but closed for lack of patient accrual. Suramin has been shown to inhibit release of CEA;[64] that perhaps it has a similar effect on PSA has recently been reported.[65] Thus, the use of PSA as a clinical trial end point needs prospective validation. In addition, the percentage of decrease that has clinical significance is unknown in hormone-refractory disease. We have evaluated the effect on the PSA assay of suramin at a concentration of 250 μg/ml. Samples with known PSA in the range of 100-2,000 μg/ml showed no differences in measured PSA values with or without suramin.[65]

Examination of reported results in several centers does show that suramin has activity in this disease and that future studies are warranted. It also provides the rationale for investigating suramin in combination. In vitro studies have shown synergy with Adriamycin and tumor necrosis factor at concentrations that are well below those associated with significant toxicities.[67] Further, the lower limit, 200 μg/ml, may be different for different tumor types. A lower concentration range may improve patient tolerance.

The actions of suramin are not restricted to growth factor inhibition, as suramin has a variety of effects. As previously noted, these actions include inhibition of glycosaminoglycan synthesis, glycolysis, and protein kinase C. The effects of angiogenesis and cell motility also have been reported.[30] Suramin represents the first of a class of compounds. As mechanisms are understood, analogues with a wider therapeutic index can be designed. However, because one action of suramin is growth factor inhibition, one must recognize that treatment can do harm. As noted in several cell systems, suramin may block inhibitory growth factors that may accelerate tumor growth. Ultimately, more specific treatments will reflect a better understanding of prostate cancer biology and the complex interaction of prostate epithelial cells and the surrounding stroma. This may allow prospective identification of tumors that may be sensitive to this type of therapy.

References

1. WHO Technical Report Series #247. WHO Expert Committee on Trypanosomiasis. 1st report. Geneva, 1962.
2. Hawking F. Suramin: with special reference to onchocerciasis. Adv Pharmacol Chemother 1978; 15:189-322.
3. De Clercq E. Suramin: a potent inhibitor of the reverse transcriptase of RNA tumor viruses. Cancer Lett 1979; 8:9-22.
4. Mitsuya H, Popovic M, Yarchoan R, et al. Suramin protection of T cells in vitro against infectivity and cytopathic effect of HTLV-III. Science 1984; 226:172-74.
5. Williams L, Tremble P, Lavin M, et al. Platelet-derived growth factor receptors form a high affinity state in membrane preparations. J Biol Chem 1984; 259:5287-94.
6. Ashby H, DiMattina M, Linehan M, et al. The inhibition of human adrenal steroidogenic enzyme activities by suramin. J Clin Endocrinol Metabol 1989; 68:505-08.
7. Coffey RJ, Leof EB, Shipley GD, et al. Suramin inhibition of growth factor receptor binding and mitogenicity in AKR-2B cells. J Cell Physiol 1987; 132:143-48.
8. Berns EMJJ, Schurmans ALG, Bolt J, et al. Antiproliferative effects of suramin on androgen responsive tumour cells. Eur J Cancer 1990; 26:470-74.
9. Pollak M, Richard M. Suramin blockade of insulinlike growth factor I-stimulated proliferation of human osteosarcoma cells. JNCI 1990; 82:1349-52.
10. Hosang M. Suramin binds to platelet-derived growth factor and inhibits its biological activity. J Cell Biochem 1985; 29:265-73.
11. Knabbe C, Kellner C, Schmahl M, et al. Suramin inhibits growth of human prostate carcinoma cells by inactivation of growth factor action. Proc Amer Assoc Cancer Res 1989; 30:295.
12. Morton RA, Isaacs JT, Isaacs WB. Differential effects of growth factor antagonists on neoplastic and normal prostatic cells. The Prostate 1990: 17:327-36.
13. Davies M, Lloyd JB, Beck F. The effect of trypan blue, suramin and aurothiomalate on the breakdown of ^{125}I-labelled albumin within rat liver lysosomes. Biochem J 1971; 121:21-26.
14. Constantopoulos G, Rees S, Cragg BG, et al. Effect of suramin on degradative enzymes of sphingolipids in rats. Res Commun Chem Pathol Pharmacol 1981; 32:87-97.
15. Constantopoulos G, Rees S, Cragg BG, et al. Experimental animal model for mucopolysaccharidosis: suramin induced glycosaminoglycan and sphingolipids accumulation in rat. Proc Natl Acad Sci USA 1980; 77:3700-04.

16. Ono K, Nakara H, Fukushima M. Differential inhibition of various deoxyribonucleic and ribonucleic acid polymerases by suramin. Eur J Biochem 1988; 172:349-53.
17. Moriyana Y, Nelson N. Inhibition of vacuolar H+-ATPases by fusidic acid and suramin. FEBS LETT 1988; 234:383-86.
18. Hensey CE, Boscoboinik D, Azzi A. Suramin, an anti-cancer drug, inhibits protein kinase C and induces differentiation in neuroblastoma cell clone NB2A. FEBS LETT 1989; 258:156-58.
19. Fantini J, Rognoni JB, Roccabianca M, et al. Suramin inhibits cell growth and glycolytic activity and triggers differentiation of human colonic adenocarcinoma cell clone HT-29-D4. J Biol Chem 1989; 264-10282-86.
20. Fantini J, Verrier B, Robert C, et al. Suramin-induced differentiation of human colonic adenocarcinoma cell clone HT29-D4 in serum free medium. Exp Cell Res 1990; 89:109-17.
21. Thompson TC. Growth factors and oncogenes in prostatic cancer. Cancer Cells 1990; 2:345-54.
22. Connolly JM, Rose DP. Production of epidermal growth factor and transforming growth factor alpha by the androgen-responsive LNCaP human prostate cancer cell line. The Prostate 1990; 16:209-18.
23. Wilding G, Valverius E, Knabbe C, Gelmann EP. Role of transforming growth factor alpha in human prostate cancer cell growth. The Prostate 1989; 15:1-12.
24. Mori H, Maki M, Oishi K, et al. Increased expression of genes for fibroblast growth factor and transforming growth factor β-2 in human benign prostatic hyperplasia. Prostate 1990; 13:241-247.
25. Mydlo JH, Bulbul MA, Richon VM, et al. Heparin-binding growth factor isolated from human prostatic extracts. The Prostate 1988; 12:343-355.
26. Mydlo JH, Michaeli J, Heston WDW, Fair WR. Expression of basic fibroblast growth factor mRNA in benign prostatic hyperplasia and prostatic carcinoma. Prostate 1988; 13:241-47.
27. Story MT, Sasse J, Jacobs SC, Lawson RK. Prostatic growth factor: purification and structural relationship to basic fibroblast growth factor. Biochemistry 1987; 26:3843-49.
28. Mansson PE, Adams P, Kan M, McKeehan WL. Heparin-binding growth factor gene expression and receptor characteristics in normal rat prostate and two transplantable rat prostate tumors. Cancer Res 1989; 49:2485-94.
29. Nishi N, Matuo Y, Wada F. Partial purification of a major type of rat prostatic growth factors: characterization as an epidermal growth factor relative mitogen. The Prostate 1988; 13:209-220.
30. Pienta KJ, Isaacs WB, Vindivich D, Coffey DS. The effects of basic fibroblast growth factor and suramin on cell motility and growth on rat prostate cancer cells. J Urol 1991; 145:199-202.
31. Hofer DR, Sherwood ER, Bromberg WD, et al. The functional role of transforming growth factor alpha as an autocrine growth factor in androgen-independent human prostatic carcinoma. Cancer Res 1991; 51:2780-85.
32. Sandgren EP, Luetteke RD, Palmiter RL, et al. Overexpression of TGF- α in transgenic mice: induction of epithelial hyperplasia, pancreatic metaplasia and carcinoma of the breast. Cell 1990; 61:1121-35.
33. Kim JH, Sherwood ER, Krengel SS, Kozlowski JM. Cytostatic and cytotoxic effects of suramin on human prostate cancer cell lines, PC3 and DU145. J Urol 1990; 143:213.
34. Ewing MW, LaRocca R, Stein CA, et al. Effect of suramin on proliferation of human prostate carcinoma. Proc Amer Assoc Cancer Res 1989; 30:310.
35. Heston WDW, Fair WR, Huryk R, Russo P. Growth inhibitory effect of suramin on urologic tumors in vitro. J Urol 1989; 141:352A (729).
36. Scher H, Heston WDW. Suramin as an archetypical compound for the development of growth factor antagonists in the treatment of genitourinary malignancies. In: Lawson H, Lepor R, eds. Genitourinary oncology. New York: Martinus Nijhoff Publishers (in press).
37. Rago R, Mitchen J, Cheng A, et al. Metabolic effects of suramin (S) on human prostate cancer cells. Proc Amer Assoc Cancer Res 1990; 31:1288.
38. Mitchen JL, Rago RP, Wilding G. Effects of suramin and TGFβ on the proliferation of primary epithelial culture (PEC) for normal, benign hyperplastic (BPH) and cancerous human prostates. Proc Amer Assoc Cancer Res 1990; 31:1289.
39. Martikainen P, Kyprianou N, Isaacs JT. Effect of transforming growth factor-β_1 on proliferation and death of rat prostatic cells. Endocrinology 1990; 127:2963-68.

40. Stein CA, LaRocca R, McAtee N, et al. Suramin - an anti-cancer drug with a unique mechanism of action. J Clin Oncol 1988; 7:499-508.
41. Stein CA, LaRocca R, Myers C. Suramin. an old compound with new biology. Principles and Practice of Oncology, May 1990.
42. Cooper M, LaRocca R, Stein C, Myers C. Pharmacokinetic monitoring is necessary for the safe use of suramin as an anticancer drug. Proc Amer Assoc Cancer Res 1989; 30:242 (963).
43. Forrest A, Scher HI, Tong W, et al. Development of an adaptive control algorithm for suramin. Proc Am Soc Clin Oncol 1990; 9:73 (abst 284).
44. Drusano GL, Forrest A, Snyder MJ, Reed MD, Blumer JL. An evaluation of optimal sampling strategy and adaptive study design. Clin Pharmacol Ther 1988; 44:232-38.
45. Van Oosterom AT, De Simedt EA, Denis JJ, et al. Suramin for prostatic cancer: a phase I/II study in advanced extensively pretreated disease. Eur J Cancer 1990; 26:422.
46. Pinedo H, van Rijswijk REN (Vu Academisch Ziekenhuis, Amsterdam). Personal communication, 1990.
47. Tong WP, Scher HI, Petrylak DP, et al. A rapid assay of suramin in plasma. J Liqud Chromatogr 1990; 13:2269-84.
48. LaRocca RV, Meer J, Gilliat RW, et al. Suramin-induced polyneuropathy. Neurology 1990; 40:954-60.
49. Horne MV, Stein CY, La Rocca RV, Myers CE. Circulating glycosaminoglycans anticoagulants associated with suramin treatment. Blood 1988; 71:273-79.
50. Weiss GH, Janis-Dow CA, Cooper MR, Linehan WM, Myers CE. Phamacokinetics and biodistribution of suramin. J Urol 1990; 143:218 (243A).
51. Holland EJ, Stein CA, Palestine AG, et al. Suramin keratopathy. Amer J Opthalmol 1988; 106:216-221.
52. Senderowicz A, Scher H, Gordon M, et al. Infectious complications of suramin in patients with genitourinary tumors. Proc Amer Assoc Cancer Res 1991; 32:203(1213).
53. Ahmann FR, Schwartz J, Dorr R, Salmon S. Suramin in hormone resistant metastatic prostate cancer: significant anticancer activity but unanticipated toxicity. Proc Amer Soc Clin Oncol 1991; 10:178(574).
54. Christian M. T89-0084. Phase II trial of suramin in hormone refractory prostatic cancer. Personal communication, 1991.
55. Myers CE, Stein C, LaRocca R, Cooper M, Cassidy J, McAtee N. Suramin: an antagonist of heparin-binding tumor growth factors with activity against a broad spectrum of human tumors. Proc Amer Soc Clin Oncol 1989; 8:66 (256).
56. Myers CE, LaRocca R, Stein C, et al. Treatment of hormonally refractory prostate cancer with suramin. Proc Amer Soc Clin Oncol 1990; 9:133 (517).
57. Dawson N. Walter Reed Medical Center. Personal communication, 1990.
58. Armand JP, Droz JP. Institute Gustave-Roussy. Personal communication, 1991.
59. Eisenberger M, Jodrell D, Sinibaldi V, et al. Preliminary evidence of anti-tumor activity against prostate cancer (PrCa) observed in a phase I trial with suramin. Proc Amer Soc Clin Oncol 1991; 10:168(537).
60. Iversen J, Scher H, Motzer R, et al. Suramin (SUR): impact of individualized pharmacokinetics (PK) dosing on outcome in patients with prostatic cancer (PC) and renal cell carinoma (RCC). Proc Amer Soc Clin Oncol 10 1991; 10:103(283).
61. Petrylak DP, Scher HI, Li Z, Curley T, Geller N. Prognostic factors for survival of patients treated with single-agent chemotherapy bidimensionally measurable hormone refractory metastatic prostatic cancer. Proc Amer Assoc Cancer Res 1990; 31:225 (abstr 1336).
62. Gerber GS, Choak GW. Prostate specific antigen for assessing response to ketoconazole and prednisone in patients with hormone refractory prostate cancer. J Urol 1990; 144:1177-79.
63. Tannock I, Gospodarowicz M, Meakin W, Panzarella T, Stewart L, Rider W. Treatment of metastatic prostatic cancer with low-dose prednisone: evaluation of pain and quality of life as pragmatic indices of response. J Clin Oncol 1990; 7:590-97.
64. Fantini J, Rognoni J-B, Theveniau M, et al. Impaired carcinoembryonic antigen release during the process of suramin-induced differentiation of the human colic adenocarcinoma cell clone HT29-D4. J Cell Physiol 1990; 143:468-74.

65. LaRocca RV, Danesi R, Cooper MR, et al. Effects of suramin on human prostate cancer cells in vitro. J Urol 1991; 145:393-98.
66. Scher HI, Nisselbaum J. Unpublished observations, 1990.
67. Freuhof JP, Myers CE, Sinha BK. Synergistic activity of suramin with tumor necrosis factor α and doxorubicin on human prostate cancer cell lines. JNCI 1990; 82:1206-09.
68. Rapoport BL, Ansell S, Coccia-Portugal MA, et al. Phase II clinical study of suramin in combination with mitomycin-C in patients with hormone refractory prostate cancer. Proc Amer Soc Clin Oncol 1991; 10:177(573).

11

EVIDENCE FOR A GENE INVOLVED IN THE ORIGIN OF HUMAN RENAL CELL CARCINOMA

W. Marston Linehan, M.D.

IN THE EARLY 1970s, Knudson suggested that there may be a recessive oncogene or tumor suppressor gene asssociated with the initiation of some forms of cancer.[1] In 1979, a pedigree was reported of a familial form of renal cell carcinoma in which the renal cell carcinoma was associated with a karyotypic abnormality of a translocation between the short arm of chromosome 3 and chromosome 8.[2] Subsequently, in 1982, Pathak and co-workers reported a second family with renal cell carcinoma in which there was a chromosome 3 to chromosome 11 translocation.[3] These 2 studies provided evidence that there may be a linkage between a structural change in chromosome 3 in hereditary as well as sporadic renal cell carcinoma.

DNA Sequence Deletion Identified

These observations led to a search for a DNA sequence deletion on the short arm of chromosome 3 in sporadic renal cell carcinoma by use of a molecular technique called restriction fragment polymorphism analysis (RFLP). A DNA sequence deletion, suggesting the presence of a tumor suppressor or antioncogene, was identified on the short arm of chromosome 3 in tissue from 11/11 evaluable patients with a sporadic form of renal cell carcinoma.[4] Subsequent studies have been performed in which tumor tissue from other patients with sporadic renal cell carcinoma has been analyzed for DNA sequence deletions at the 3p14-21 region, and deletions have been observed in most.

We have currently evaluated tissue from 60 patients with advanced renal cell carcinoma with 10 polymorphic probes localized to the short arm of chromosome 3. Fifty-eight of the 60 patients were evaluable (heterozygous) for at least one of the polymorphic probes localized to chromosome 3. There was evidence for loss of heterozygosity in 51 of 58 patients (88%). We found DNA sequence deletions at this location in patients with both localized as well as advanced disease. When we analyzed whether or not there would be loss of heterozygosity on the short arm of chromosome 3 in a "benign" renal tumor, oncocytoma (i.e., whether or not loss of heterozygosity on chromosome 3 was associated with a benign tumor of the kidney), we found no evidence for loss of heterozygosity.[5]

We have also analyzed regions on chromosomes 11, 13, and 17 for loss of heterozygosity. We have found DNA sequence deletions at these other chromosomal locations in tissue from some patients with advanced (stage IV) disease; however, we have not identified deletions in patients with stage I/II renal cell carcinoma, suggesting that the abnormalities on chromosome 11, 13, and 17 may be associated with disease progression.

Linkage with von Hippel-Lindau Disease

These observations raise the possibility that there is a gene located on chromosome 3p involved in the pathogenesis of renal cell carcinoma. These observations are supported by recent observations in von Hippel-Lindau disease (VHL). Von Hippel-Lindau disease is a rare hereditary illness that is inherited as an autosomal dominant trait. Individuals who inherit the disease gene have a predisposition to develop retinal angiomas, spinal and cerebellar hemangioblastomas, pheochromocytomas, renal and pancreatic cysts, cystadenomas of the epididymis, and renal cell carcinomas. Renal cell carcinomas in patients with VHL are characterized by early age of onset, bilaterality, and multiplicity. Seizinger et al have reported that the VHL gene is located on chromosome 3p.[6] We examined renal cell carcinomas associated with VHL for chromosome 3p allele loss because of the location of the VHL gene, reports of chromosome 3p alterations in tumors of this type, and previous findings of consistent 3p allele loss in sporadic renal cell carcinoma. Examination of renal cell carcinomas from patients with VHL may resolve the issue of whether chromosome 3p allele loss in renal tumors reflects a genetic change important in the origin or evolution of these tumors.

When we analyzed renal cell carcinomas from patients with VHL, all renal cell carcinomas had a loss of chromosome 3p alleles. There was also a pattern to 3p allele loss in hereditary renal cell carcinomas. Multiple renal cell carcinomas in individual patients with VHL showed loss of the same chromosome 3p alleles, demonstrating that the same chromosome was deleted in each tumor.[7] In the hereditary renal cell carcinomas that could be examined for maternal or paternal origin of 3p alleles, the chromosome 3p alleles that were lost were located on the chromosome 3 bearing the wild-type allele of the VHL gene.[7] These observations indicate that the loss of the balancing wild-type allele of the VHL gene may be a prerequisite for tumorigenesis in renal cell carcinoma associated with VHL. Recent studies by our group have (1) confirmed by linkage analysis that the VHL gene is located on the short arm of chromosome 3 and (2) demonstrated its association to a highly polymorphic marker located at 3p26, distal to cRAF1.

Conclusion

This work indicates that there may be a least one gene located on chromosome 3p that is associated with renal cell carcinoma and strongly suggests that the mechanism of formation of renal cell carcinoma involves inactivation of both copies of this renal cell carcinoma gene. Further studies are currently underway to identify this tumor suppressor gene involved in the development of sporadic as well as familial renal cell carcinoma and to provide further understanding of its function in order to lead to the development of more effective means of treating this disease.

References

1. Knudson AG Jr. Mutation and cancer: statistical study of retinoblastoma. Proc Natl Acad Sci USA 1971; 68:820-23.
2. Cohen AJ, Li FP, Berg S, et al. Hereditary renal-cell carcinoma associated with a chromosomal translocation. N Engl J Med 1979; 301: 592-95.
3. Pathak S, Strong LC, Ferrell RE, Trindade A. Familial renal cell carcinoma with a 3;11 chromosome translocation limited to tumor cells. Science 1982; 217:939-41.
4. Zbar B, Brauch H, Talmadge C, Linehan M. Loss of alleles of loci on the short arm of chromosome 3 in renal cell carcinoma. Nature 1987; 327:721-24.
5. Brauch H, Tory K, Linehan WM, Weaver DJ, Lovell MA, Zbar B. Molecular analysis of the short arm of chromosome 3 in five renal oncocytomas. J Urol 1990; 143: 622-24.
6. Seizinger BR, Rouleau GA, Ozelius LJ, et al. Von Hippel-Lindau disease maps to the region of chromosome 3 associated with renal cell carcinoma. Nature 1988; 332: 268-69.
7. Tory K, Brauch H, Linehan M, et al. Specific genetic change in tumors associated with von Hippel-Lindau disease. JNCI 1989; 81: 1097-1101.

12

SURGICAL APPROACHES TO THE TREATMENT OF RENAL CELL CARCINOMA

Andrew Novick, M.D.

SURGERY REMAINS THE MOST effective method of treatment for patients with renal cell carcinoma (RCC). Radical nephrectomy provides optimum curative therapy for patients with localized RCC and an anatomically and functionally normal opposite kidney. The therapeutic value of performing a regional lymphadenectomy is controversial. The 5-yr survival rate following radical nephrectomy for a stage I RCC is 60-70%. This rate is reduced in the presence of perinephric fat involvement (50-60%), renal vein involvement (50-60%), vena caval involvement (25-50%), extension to regional lymph nodes (5-30%), invasion of adjacent organs (0-5%), and distant metastases (0-5%).

Conservative Surgery Increasingly Used

Conservative or nephron-sparing surgery is being increasingly used in the management of RCC due to excellent reported long-term survival rates, improved surgical techniques, and the increasing discovery of incidental RCCs upon noninvasive imaging studies. Current data indicate that conservative surgery provides effective therapy for patients with localized RCC in whom preservation of renal function is a relevant clinical consideration. This includes patients with localized RCC and a functioning opposite kidney when that kidney is involved with a disorder (e.g., calculi, diabetes, pyelonephritis, nephrosclerosis) that might cause future progressive renal functional impairment. The technical success rate with nephron-sparing surgery is excellent, and long-term patient survival free of cancer is comparable to that obtained after radical nephrectomy, particularly for stage I RCC. The major disadvantage of conservative surgery is the associated 10% risk of local tumor recurrence in the operated kidney. The risk of local recurrence after radical nephrectomy has not been determined, but is presumably much less.

Current controversy exists concerning the role of a conservative operation in patients with unilateral RCC and a normal opposite kidney with no intercurrent condition that subsequently might impair the function of that kidney. A nephron-sparing operation is being performed in some of these patients with small peripheral RCCs, particularly those that are discovered incidentally. To date, the value of a conservative operation in this setting is not established, and radical nephrectomy still must be considered the treatment of choice.

Surgical Removal of IVC Thrombus

Involvement of the inferior vena cava (IVC) increases the technical difficulty of performing radical nephrectomy for RCC. For patients with nonmetastatic RCC and IVC involvement, 5-yr survival rates of 47-68% have been reported following complete surgical excision. The presence of lymph node or distant metastasis in such cases carries a dismal prognosis that is not appreciably altered by radical surgical extirpation. Accurate preoperative information regarding the presence and complete extent of an IVC tumor thrombus is essential to determine the appropriate operative approach. Although inferior vena cavography has been the most accurate diagnostic study for assessment of IVC thrombi, recent data indicate that magnetic resonance imaging is an equally accurate and less invasive method. Renal arteriography remains a useful preoperative study, since many caval thrombi demonstrate hypervascularity with distinct arterial supply from the renal artery. When this finding is observed, preoperative renal arterial embolization can facilitate surgical removal of the thrombus.

In performing surgical removal of an IVC thrombus, it is essential to obtain control of the cava above the thrombus to prevent intraoperative embolization of a tumor fragment. Several techniques have been used to remove large caval thrombi when distal caval control cannot be achieved below the liver. Cardiopulmonary bypass (CBP) with deep hypothermic circulatory arrest (DHCA) offers several important advantages in this setting. From 1984 to 1989, 43 patients with a suprahepatic or intrahepatic vena caval tumor thrombus from renal cell carcinoma underwent surgical treatment with CPB and DHCA. The operative mortality rate was 4.7%, and the incidence of major postoperative complications was 30.2%. No ischemic or neurologic complications arose, and no cases of perioperative tumor embolization were encountered. The 3-yr survival rate in patients with localized RCC was 63.9%. These data indicate that CPB with DHCA is a safe and effective approach.

Metastatic Renal Cell Carcinoma

Surgery plays a palliative role in some patients with metastatic RCC who are experiencing severe disability from associated local symptoms, although some patients in this category can be managed with angioinfarction. In patients with RCC and a solitary resectable metastasis, surgical excision is warranted based on reported 5-yr survival rates of 30-35%. Many biologic response modifier protocols to treat patients with metastatic RCC currently require preliminary removal of the primary tumor; however, the advantage of nephrectomy in this setting has not been established.

Bibliography

1. Novick AC, Streem S, Montie JE, et al. Conservative surgery for renal cell carcinoma: A single center experience with 100 patients. J Urol 1989; 141:835.
2. Montie JE, Jackson CL, Cosgrove D, Streem S, Novick AC. Resection of large inferior vena caval thrombi from renal cell carcinoma with the use of circulatory arrest. J Urol 1988; 139:25.
3. Welch M, Bazaral MG, Schmidt R, Cosgrove I, Montie J, Novick AC. Anesthetic management for surgical removal of renal cell carcinoma with caval or atrial tumor thrombus using deep hypothermic circulatory arrest. J Cardiothoracic Anesthesia 1989; 3:580.
4. Spencer W, Novick AC, et al. Surgical treatment of localized renal cell carcinoma in von Hippel Lindau disease. J Urol 1988; 139:50.
5. Maatman TJ, Novick AC, et al. Renal oncocytoma: a diagnostic dilemma. J Urol 1984; 132:878.

13

NEW APPLICATIONS OF BIOLOGIC THERAPY

Michael T. Lotze, M.D., F.A.C.S.

Interleukin-2 as a Pharmacologic Reagent

A VARIETY OF BOTH immunologic as well as toxic effects are associated with the administration of interleukin-2 (IL-2). The earliest effect noted following IL-2 administration is a rapid decrease in circulating lymphokine-activated killer (LAK) cell precursors, which is noted within minutes following a dose of IL-2. Within 2 hr following a dose of IL-2, the heart rate increases and mean arterial blood pressure and systemic vascular resistance decrease, with nadirs occurring at about 4 hr following the dose of IL-2. Within 2 hr after administration of IL-2, patients untreated with antipyretics develop chills and within 3-4 hr develop fever. Increases in serum ACTH (to levels as high as 150-200 mg/ml) are noted at 4 hr, and subsequent increases of cortisol to levels as high as 30-50 μg/dl are noted at 5-6 hr.

With continued treatment with IL-2, a variety of hematologic and systemic effects are noted. We usually administer 30,000-100,000 Cetus U/kg of IL-2 3 times a day. With this regimen, profound lymphopenia is noted within 4 hr and is maintained throughout IL-2 administration. When IL-2 is stopped, a rebound in peripheral lymphocytes numbers to 2-16–fold greater levels than those observed prior to treatment is noted. Similarly, a marked increase in the number of circulating cells bearing the IL-2 receptor (Tac) amounting to as many as 30% of cells is noted. Myocardial depression as measured by decreased ejection fraction is observed in most patients, as also are profound cholestasis and prerenal azotemia associated with marked sodium reabsorption. Many of the clinical findings are related to the development of a vascular leak syndrome. Serum levels of gamma interferon, tumor necrosis factor, and IL-6 are detectable within 2-6 hr of IL-2 administration. Many of the findings related to IL-2 treatment are likely due to the secondary elaboration of these and other cytokines.

The antitumor effects of IL-2 are usually manifested by a slow decrease in tumor size, first noted at 1-2 mo following treatment. In some patients, changes in the size of cutaneous melanoma nodules has been noted as early as 3-4 days after therapy is begun. The histologic examination of these sites reveal marked induction of DR expression on tumor cells, as well as tumor-infiltrating lymphoctyes in virtually all regressing lesions that we have examined.

Combination with Other Lymphokines

Based on biologic principles developed in vitro and subsequently extended to murine tumor models, combination lymphokine protocols have been proposed and developed in humans. Very similarly to the stepwise development of cancer chemotherapy in which combinations of individual agents were found to be effective and combinations were employed to develop more potent therapeutic regimens, combinations of lymphokines have been employed in humans. In studies performed in mice, combinations of tumor necrosis factor (TNF) and IL-2 were found to be markedly synergistic when assessing regression of tumor, prolongation of survival, or improved cure rates when compared with either agent alone. These findings occurred only in immunogenic tumors and not in nonimmunogenic tumors. Although these combination studies were quite convincing in our murine models,[2,5] treatment with TNF and IL-2 in our clinical protocols have yet to convincingly demonstrate benefit when compared to IL-2 alone.

The in vivo activity of IL-2 in conjunction with interferon alpha was first demonstrated in murine metastases models.[4] Synergy that was observed in tumors within the liver appeared to be related to the induction of asialo GM-1 positive cells, which are a marker of the large granular lymphocytes that mediate NK (natural killer), LAK, and lymphocyte-directed antibody-dependent cell-mediated cytotoxicity (ADCC) activity. We have demonstrated similar effects in murine models using methylcolanthrene-induced sarcomas. In this setting, synergy was noted only with immunogenic tumors. Based on these studies, clinical trials have now been performed in more than 105 patients with combinations of alpha interferon and IL-2. As predicted by our murine models, there is additive toxicity with alpha interferon with both neurologic and hemodynamic effects being limiting and possibly increased efficacy at highest doses employed.

Combination with Monoclonal Antibodies

In murine models, combinations of specific antitumor monoclonal antibodies have been effective in treatment of both B16 melanoma and lymphomas, using anti-idiotypic antibodies. We have treated more than 50 patients with combinations of monoclonal antibodies and IL-2, with total cumulative doses of antibody as high as 6 gm/m^2 administered in conjunction with therapeutic doses of IL-2 at 100,000 U/kg. Only modest antitumor effects have been observed in 2 patients. We plan to assess antibodies that have more potent ADCC activity. In addition, we plan to combine the adoptive transfer of LAK cells with IL-2 and the L6 monoclonal antibody with the hope of mimicking similar successful strategies in murine models. In our earliest studies of IL-2 in conjunction with murine monoclonal antibodies, prolonged whole body retention as measured by the use of radiolabeled monoclonal antibodies was noted.[5]

Interleukin-4 Studies

We have recently evaluated the novel T cell growth factor now known as interleukin-4 and its ability to generate cells with LAK activity in murine models and, more recently, in human studies.[6] Recombinant murine IL-4 induces significant LAK activity from resting murine splenocytes. Recombinant IL-4 clearly suppresses LAK activity from resting human cells treated with IL-2, however. Most interestingly, a subsequent 3-day incubation with IL-4 following a brief 24-hr exposure to IL-2 allowed the induction of potent LAK activity, and, at one unit of IL-2, appeared to further synergize in the induction of this activity.

We have examined a group of patients receiving IL-2 in vivo and have been able to confirm that cells obtained from the peripheral blood of such recently treated patients are capable of generating LAK activity when stimulated with IL-4 alone in vitro. We have used IL-4 in conjunction with IL-2 to grow tumor-infiltrating lymphocytes (TILs) directly from melanoma. Growth of TILs with IL-2 and IL-4 not only increases the total number of cells obtained but also decreases the nonspecific cytolytic activity. The importance of IL-4 in response to murine tumors has recently been demonstrated.[7]

Based on these studies, we have initiated clinical protocols using IL-4 alone in a phase 1 trial. We have treated a total of 60 patients with IL-4 for a total of up to 15 doses with toxicites of a vascular leak syndrome, gastritis, and vasal congestion. Combination protocols with IL-2 have begun.

Adoptive Therapy with Tumor-Infiltrating Lymphocytes

Initial studies from our group indicated that TILs grown from murine tumors and expanded in recombinant IL-2 were 50- to 100-fold more active in adoptive transfer than LAK cells.[8] In these studies, it was clear that the cells were most efficacious in the setting of immunosuppression with either irradiation or cyclophosphamide.

Combinations of IL-2 with expanded TILs are being evaluated in humans. We have developed culture techniques that allow us to expand large numbers of TILs and are currently treating patients with a planned 10^{11} cells or greater. We have now treated more than 100 patients with IL-2 and TILs.[9] Current studies examine preparation of TILs with IL-4 as well as IL-2 for use in adoptive immunotherapy.

Gene Transfer Mediated by Cultured TILs

One of the major problems with the development of adoptive immunotherapy with TILs has been our inability to follow these cells for prolonged periods after administration. Because of this, the in vivo conditions required for their growth and antitumor effects are difficult to define. The use of retroviral vectors for introducing genes into mammalian cells has been developed for correction of a variety of different genetic disorders and, in particular, the adenosine deaminase deficiency syndrome. We have recently adopted these techniques for marking TILs with incompetent retroviral vectors containing a gene that confers resistance to the neomycin analogue G418. These cells can be selected in vitro and used as tagged cells on transfer into patients to allow their ready identification through use of a variety of different techniques.[10] To date, 6 patients have received such cells.

References

1. Lotze MT, Rosenberg SA. Interleukin-2 as a pharmacologic reagent. In: Smith EK, Interleukin-2. Orlando: Academic Press, 1988; 237-94.
2. Asher A, Mule JJ, Reichert CM, Shiloni E, Rosenberg SA. Studies on the antitumor efficacy of systemically administered recombinant tumor necrosis factor against several murine tumors in vivo. J. Immunol 1987; 138:963-74.
3. McIntosh JK, Mule JJ, Merino MJ, Rosenberg SA. Synergistic antitumor effects of immunotherapy with recombinant interleukin-2 and recombinant tumor necrosis factor. Cancer Res 1988; 48:4011-17.
4. Brunda MJ, Bellantoni D, Sulich V. In vivo anti-tumor activity of combinations of interferon alpha and interleukin-2 in a murine model. Correlation of efficacy with the induction of cytotoxic cells resembling natural killer cells. Int J Cancer 1987; 40:365-71.
5. Lotze MT, Rosenberg SA. The immunologic treatment of cancer. CA 1988; 38:69-64.
6. Kawakami Y, Rosenberg SA, Lotze, MT. Interleukin-4 promotes the growth of tumor-infiltrating lymphocytes cytotoxic for human autologous melanoma. J Exp Med 1988; 168:2183-91.
7. Kern DE, Peace DJ, Klarnet JP, Cheever MA, Greenberg PD. IL-4 is an endogenous T cell growth factor during the immune response to a syngeneic retrovirus-induced tumor. J Immunol 1988; 141:2824-30.
8. Rosenberg SA, Spiess P, Lafreniere R. A new approach to the adoptive immunotherapy of cancer with tumor-infiltrating lymphocytes. Science 1986; 233:1318-21.
9. Rosenberg SA, Packard B, Aebersold PM, et al. Immunotherapy of patients with metastatic melanoma using tumor infiltrating lymphocytes and interleukin-2: Preliminary report. N Engl J Med 1988; 319:1676-80.
10. Kasid A, Morecki S, Aebersold PM, et al. Human gene transfer: Characterization of human tumor-infiltrating lymphocytes as vehicles for retroviral-mediated gene transfer in man. Proc Natl Acad Sci 1990; 87:473-77.

14

CARCINOGENESIS IN EXPERIMENTAL BLADDER CANCER

Ryoichi Oyasu, M.D.

SUPERFICIAL BLADDER TUMOR COMPRISES about 70-80% of bladder cancer cases, and progression to muscle-invasive carcinoma occurs in 10-15% of patients with superficial disease. Of patients presenting with muscle-invasive cancer, 70-80% do not have a history of superficial disease.

Most human bladder cancers are papillary transitional carcinoma of low malignant potential and characteristically recur following endoscopic resection. However, about 20-30% of bladder cancer patients present initially with a deeply invasive, potentially lethal carcinoma. Another deeply invasive type of bladder cancer is squamous carcinoma, which is uncommon in the Western world.

Experimental and clinical evidence suggests that bladder carcinogenesis is a multifactorial and multistage process that includes initiation, promotion, and progression. Some industrial chemicals have been identified as bladder carcinogens, and cigarette smoking has been shown to increase the risk of bladder cancer. Recent studies in both human and experimental animals have indicated that most urothelial carcinomas arise in a generalized "field" change where the entire epithelium is involved in the carcinogenic process and that endoscopically visible neoplasms represent only the most florid components.

The mechanism or mechanisms underlying the development of bladder carcinomas remain unclear. We believe that the high rate of tumor recurrence (new growths) stems from the preferential response of carcinogen-initiated cells to growth-promoting effects exhibited by urinary growth factors, notably the epidermal growth factor (EGF).[1] One of our recent studies clearly supports this hypothesis.[2] The recurrent tumors are almost always low-grade, noninvasive papillary lesions similar to the primary tumors. Thus, growth factors of urine do not appear responsible for progression of the disease to higher-grade carcinomas.

In my view, the development of deeply invasive carcinoma is due to additional genetic mutation(s) in a noninvasive carcinoma. This hypothesis is well supported by a series of experiments conducted in my laboratory using the unique animal model, the heterotopically transplanted rat urinary bladder (HTB) system.[3,4]

Separately, an in vitro system has been developed with which conversion from noninvasive to lung-metastatic carcinomas can be induced; 17 such clones have been established from a low-grade noninvasive rat urinary bladder carcinoma cell line, D44c, after in vitro treatment with N-methyl-N-nitrosourea.[5] One of our recent investigations with this in vitro system has led to the suggestion that EGF is involved in the growth of nontumorigenic transformed cells, whereas transforming growth factor α mediates the growth of tumorigenic invasive carcinoma, probably by an autocrine mechanism.[6] These clonally derived cell lines provide a useful model to study the molecular mechanism(s) involved in the conversion of noninvasion bladder carcinomas to metastasizing ones.

References

1. Yura Y, Hayashi O, Kelly M, Oyasu R. Identification of epidermal growth factor as a component of the rat urinary bladder tumor-enhancing urinary fractions. Cancer Res 1989; 49:1548-53.
2. Momose H, Kakinuma H, Oyasu R. Tumor promoting effect of urinary epidermal growth factor and transferrin in rat urinary bladder carcinogenesis. Proc Am Assoc Cancer Res 1991; 32:152.
3. Samma S, Oyasu R. Conversion from low-grade to high-grade of rat urinary bladder carcinomas. Cancer Res 1988; 48:1265-69.
4. Miyata Y, Babaya K, Oyasu R. Carcinogenesis in heterotopically-transplanted urinary bladder by N-methyl-N-nitrosourea: a model for initiation and promotion. Carcinogenesis 1981; 2:495-97.
5. Azuma M, Oyasu R. In vitro malignant conversion of low-grade rat urinary bladder carcinoma cells by exposure to N-methyl-N-nitrosourea. Cancer Res 1990; 50:7062-67.
6. Azuma M, Oyasu R. Role of epidermal growth factor and transforming growth factor α in in vitro rat urinary bladder carcinoma cell growth. Proc Am Assoc Cancer Res 1991; 32:44.

15

PHOTODYNAMIC THERAPY FOR BLADDER CANCER

Bryan P. Shumaker, M.D., F.A.C.S.

THE TREATMENT OF NONINVASIVE bladder carcinoma using dinematoporphyrin ether (DHE) and laser photodynamic therapy (PDT) is described herein. Patients treated with this modality have had positive cytology and biopsy-proven transitional cell carcinoma, no histologic evidence of muscle or prostatic urethral invasion, and negative excretory urograms.

Eighteen patients with refractory carcinoma *in situ* (Tis) have been treated, with follow-up of 18-66 mo. Twelve have had a complete response (CR) and 5 have recurred. Two of the patients recurred with invasive disease within 18 mo of treatment and required cystectomy. Three patients were re-treated: one has remained tumor-free at 3 yr, one recurred again and has been successfully managed via periodic Nd:YAG laser ablation, and one of the re-treated patients developed ureteral and prostatic uretheral involvement and underwent cystectomy. One patient was lost to follow-up immediately post-treatment. There have been no known deaths due to transitional cell carcinoma. It should be noted that all patients had failed at least 2 courses of intravesical chemotherapy, the later patients having failed intravesical treatment with bacille Calmette-Guérin (BCG) as well.

About 14 patients with superficial recurrent disease who had been resistant to repeated courses of intravesical chemotherapy also have been followed in this time period. Although follow-up data have been more difficult to accumulate because many patients were referred from out of state and returned to their own urologists for follow-up, results seem somewhat better in comparison with the Tis group. Additionally, we are not aware that any patients in this group progressed to cystectomy.

Photosensitivity for up to 6 wk is a known potential adverse reaction, but can be avoided completely if proper precautions are followed. Significant but spontaneously resolving morbidity includes a marked increase in urinary frequency, urgency, and occasionally hematuria, which gradually disappears after 6-12 wk. Careful placement of the fiberoptic tip in the center of the bladder, bladder distension during treatment with saline rather than water, instillation of the minimum volume required to "smooth out" the mucosa for complete bladder photoradiation, and delivered energy of 15 joule/cm^2 or less seems to prevent the more severe complications (i.e., bladder shrinkage) originally reported.

We also feel that there is increasing evidence that a heightened immune response (similar to intravesical BCG) is an additional and ultimately more important mechanism to explain the efficacy of PDT in long disease-free intervals.

It appears that PDT offers another practical treatment modality for noninvasive transitional cell carcinoma in patients refractory to standard surgical and intravesical chemotherapeutic regimens. The author is presently recommending to patients in these categories that they undergo a course of PDT prior to relinquishing to cystectomy.

Bibliography

1. Benson RC. Treatment of diffuse transitional cell carcinoma *in situ* by whole bladder hematoporphyrin derivative photodynamic therapy. J Urol 1985; 134:675-78.
2. Chodak G, Shumaker B. PDT fiberoptic placement training film, Nov 1986 (under contract from Photomedica, Inc.).
3. Dougherty TJ, Lawrence G, Kaufman JH, Boyle D, Welshaupt KR, Goldfarb A. Photoradiation in the treatment of recurrent breast carcinoma. JNCI 1979; 62:231-34.
4. Figge FHJ, Weiland GS, Mangiello LOJ. Affinity of neoplastic, embryonic, and traumitized tissues for porphrins and metalloporphyrins. Proc Soc Exp Biol Med 1948; 68:640-41.
5. Granelli SG, Diamond I, McDonagh AF, Wilson CB, Nielsen SL. Photochemotherapy of glioma cells by visible light and hematoprophyrin. Cancer Res 1975; 35:2567-70.
6. Hisazumi H, Misaki T, Miyoshi N. Photoradiation therapy of bladder tumors. J Urol 1983; 130:685.
7. Lipson RL, Baldes EJ, Olsen AM. The use of a derivative of hematoporphyrin in tumor detection. JNCI 1961; 26:1-11.
8. Nseyo U, Whalen RK, Duncan MR. Immune response following PDT for bladder cancer. SPIE monograph, vol. 1065, PDT mechanisms 1989; 66-72.
9. Novogrodsky A, Suthanthiran M, Stenzel K. Immune stimulatory properties of metalloporphyrins. J Immunol 1989; 143:3981-87.
10. Harty JI, Amin A, Weiman TJ, Tseng MT, Ackerman D, Broghamer W. Complications of whole bladder dihematoporphyrin ether PDT. J Urol 1989; 141:41-1346.

16

ADVANCES IN DIAGNOSIS AND TREATMENT OF SUPERFICIAL BLADDER CANCER

Mark Soloway, M.D.

Introduction

DIAGNOSIS OF PATIENTS WITH bladder cancer involves the workup for patients with gross and microscopic hematuria, as well as suspicion for men and women over 50 with irritative symptoms. Urinary cytology is highly accurate for detecting individuals with grade 2 or grade 3 transitional cell carcinoma; however, the urinary cytology may be normal or only suspicious for those with low-grade tumors. Office endoscopy, particularly with the use of the flexible cystoscope, has made initial diagnosis easier and more readily available in the office outpatient setting.

Once the identification of a patient with apparent superficial bladder cancer has been made, an excretory urogram is usually obtained to determine the status of the upper urinary tract and to ensure that the renal collecting system and ureter are uninvolved. The likelihood of an upper tract tumor is quite low for the individual with bladder cancer.

Following the diagnosis of transitional cell carcinoma, the initial maneuver is almost always transurethral resection. This provides histologic material for establishing the grade and the stage of the tumor or tumors. If possible, all tumors should be resected. Tumor grade is probably the most important prognostic factor.

A variety of lenses should be incorporated into the initial endoscopic evaluation, and it is important that the prostatic urethra be viewed and biopsied when there is a high-grade tumor present in the bladder. Transitional cell carcinoma of the prostatic urethra is being found with increasing incidence, probably due to the effectiveness of intravesical therapy in altering the natural history of tumors of the bladder. The presence of transitional cell carcinoma of the prostatic urethra will probably alter treatment.

Prognostic Categorization

Patients can be segregated into prognostic categories following the initial transurethral resection. Patients with grade 1, stage Ta lesions are very unlikely to have a subsequent tumor that invades muscle of the bladder. On the other hand, patients with tumors that are high grade and/or invade the lamina propria have a 30% chance of subsequently developing a muscle-invasive tumor and therefore need to be treated and monitored in an aggressive manner. Follow-up studies after the initial tumor resection thus will vary with the prognostic information gained from the first resection. Patients with low-grade and low-stage tumors are at little risk of progression and can be followed primarily by cytology with less frequent endoscopy.

Carcinoma *in situ* is important because it tends to be multifocal; because this is a high-grade malignancy, the potential for progression is high and patients require intensive management and monitoring. However, the natural history for individual patients with carcinoma *in situ* is quite variable. Patients with carcinoma *in situ* are appropriate candidates for intravesical therapy. A 3- to 6-mo trial of intravesical therapy is appropriate; however, if a positive cytology or persistence of carcinoma *in situ* on histology is apparent, the treatment approach should be altered.

Intravesical Therapy

Intravesical therapy has been shown to decrease the likelihood of subsequent tumor when delivered on a regular basis following endoscopic resection of all evident tumor (i.e., prophylaxis). Intravesical therapy is also capable of eradicating residual transitional cell carcinoma remaining in the bladder after incomplete resection (i.e., treatment).

Most treatment courses involve weekly instillations for 6-8 wk. If possible, patients should be segregated into treatment or prophylactic indication. Persistence of positive cytology indicates residual neoplasm in the bladder; thus, such patients receiving intravesical therapy are being treated for this reason. Alternatively, if all tumor has been resected and if the cytology subsequently is negative, then the primary purpose of giving intravesical therapy is prophylactic—to prevent a subsequent tumor or delay its onset.

Chemotherapy

Among the most commonly used intravesical drugs are thio-tepa, mitomycin-C (MIT), and bacille Calmette-Guérin (BCG).

Thio-tepa has been used for intravesical therapy for more than 25 yr. It is usually given in a dose of 30-60 mg in an equal volume of solution to make a concentration of 1 mg/ml. Although it may be absorbed, it is also reasonably safe in the absence of an extensive resection to give this soon after transurethral resection of bladder tumors. It is mandatory that the patient's white count and platelet count be monitored prior to each instillation to ensure that myelosuppression is not occurring as a result of this agent. Some of the data suggest that thio-tepa is more effective for low-grade than for high-grade tumors.

Mitomycin-C is another intravesical agent that has been quite successful, both for treatment and prophylaxis. Randomized trials suggest that it might be as effective as the more recently introduced agent BCG. When used for treatment of a persistent tumor, MIT usually is given at a dose of 40 mg in 40 ml of solution; when used for prophylaxis, 20 mg in 20 ml, delivered every other week, has been successfully used. Because MIT interacts so strongly with the urothelium, particularly when it has not healed following endoscopic resection, symptoms related to chemical cystitis may be diminished by waiting 7-10 days following resection before instilling the first dose of the drug.

BCG has recently been approved by the Food and Drug Administration for use in carcinoma *in situ* of the urinary bladder. Also, many studies have demonstrated its efficacy in both treatment and prophylaxis of other nonmuscle-invading tumors of the urinary bladder. A number of strains of BCG have been used, including the Montreal, Tice, Connaught, and the strains individually marketed in such countries as The Netherlands, Mexico, and Japan. BCG is less expensive than some of the other intravesical therapeutic agents.

Side effects related to BCG include fever, hematuria, and lower urinary tract irritative symptoms. These may vary with the dose of the instilled BCG, the immunocompetence of the patient, and the strain of BCG used. If delivered in such a way that it may gain access to the blood stream, severe toxicity and even death can occur.

Summary

Patients with superficial bladder cancer comprise a heterogeneous group. The urologist should be familiar with the entire spectrum of the disease and with the various prognostic factors so that therapy can be tailored to the individual patient. Factors that influence the therapeutic decision include a likelihood of tumor persistence following resection, tumor recurrence or new occurrence, and the likelihood of progression. Patients with low-grade, low-stage (Ta) tumors, be they unifocal or multifocal, are at little risk for progression and may not require intravesical therapy following initial endoscopic resection. On the other hand, patients with multifocal carcinoma *in situ* require intensive intravesical therapy and are at relatively high risk for development of a tumor that will invade the wall of the bladder.

Several intravesical agents are available, and urologists have the opportunity to prevent or delay the frequency of subsequent tumors in patients identified to be at high risk, either following initial tumor resection or after development of a recurrence.

Unfortunately, only limited prospective, randomized trials have been undertaken to compare the efficacy and toxicity of available intravesical agents. In addition to determining which agent is best in a randomized trial, further investigation is needed to determine the appropriate timing for endoscopic resection, and appropriate dose/response studies have yet to be performed.

17

CURRENT INDICATIONS AND SURGICAL ALTERNATIVES IN THE MANAGEMENT OF INVASIVE BLADDER CANCER

Randall G. Rowland, M.D., Ph.D.

THE ROLE OF SURGERY, namely cystectomy, in the management of bladder cancer is undergoing change. New treatment strategies using neoadjuvant chemotherapy, adjuvant chemotherapy, and combination chemotherapy and radiotherapy regimens are giving us reason to reexamine the role of cystectomy in the management of bladder cancer.

Currently, indications for radical cystectomy include multifocal Cis, Ta, or Tl tumors not responding to 3-6 mo of intravesicle chemotherapy; T2-3 tumors; and T4 tumors that have been clinically downstaged by neoadjuvant chemotherapy. These indications assume that the patient is otherwise a good candidate for surgery from a medical point of view.

An alternative to radical cystectomy is partial cystectomy. Special criteria must be met before the patient is considered a candidate for partial cystectomy. The patient must have a solitary Tl-3 tumor away from the trigone or bladder neck and also must have negative selective site biopsies. Only a small percentage of patients with invasive bladder tumors meet these criteria. Partial cystectomy usually offers the advantage of preservation of sexual function and normal voiding function, perhaps with the exception of a slight reduction in bladder capacity. Results in the literature report equivalent outcomes on a stage-for-stage basis comparing those patients who meet the restrictive criteria necessary for partial cystectomy and those with radical cystectomy.

The technique of an Indiana continent urinary reservoir from an ileocecal segment is shown in figure 17-1. The creation of the continence mechanism and the efferent

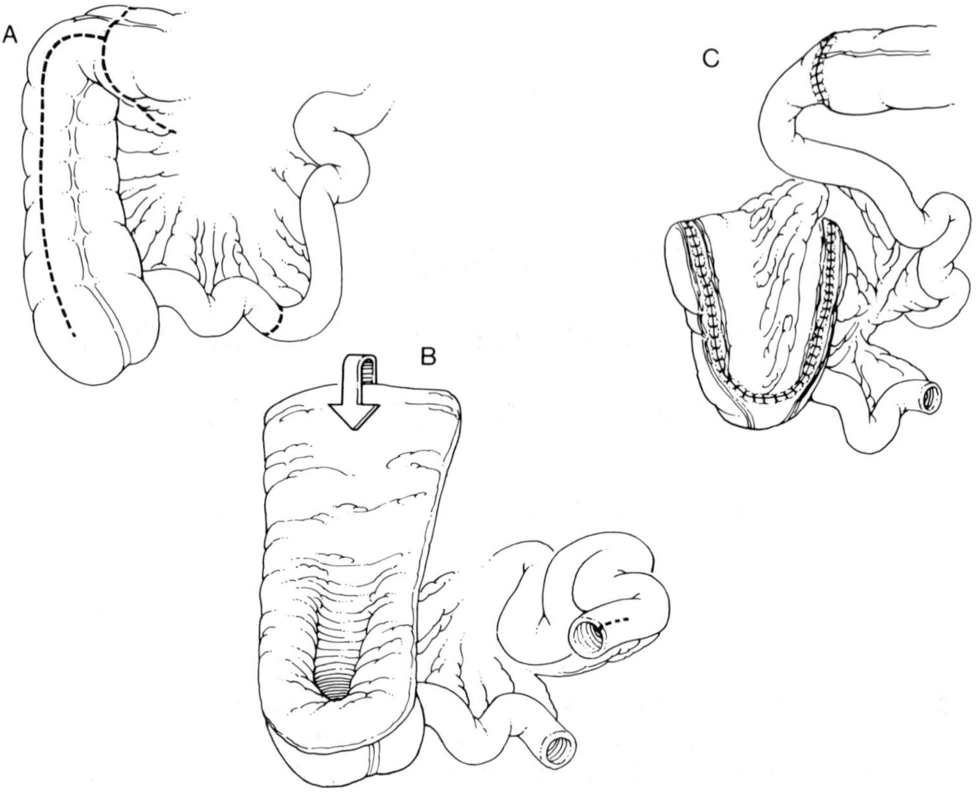

Figure 17-1. In drawing A, the dashed lines indicate incisions in the bowel and mesentery to create an ileocecal reservoir; 25-30 cm of colon and 8-10 cm of ileum are isolated. The cecum and ascending colon are opened along the antimesenteric surface to permit detubularization. In drawing B, the detubularized colonic bowel segment is folded over as indicated by the arrow. A 2-layer closure with 3-0 synthetic braided suture is performed. The completed detubularized reservoir is shown in drawing C. An ileocolostomy is performed in an end-to-end manner as shown (alternately, a stapled end-to-side anastomosis can be used). Closure of the reservoir is usually performed after completion of the efferent limb continence mechanism shown in figures 17-2 A–E.

limb is illustrated in figures 17-2A–E. Finally, the ureterocolic anastomosis is presented in figure 17-3.

Recent reports also have described optimistic results with extensive transuretheral resection of bladder tumors in carefully selected patients. Again, these patients should meet the same criteria as those having partial cystectomy, with the addition that the tumors should not be at the dome of the bladder or the trigone or bladder neck. The extensive transuretheral resection necessary to be successful at radical TUR could potentially cause problems with an intraperitoneal perforation if performed at the dome

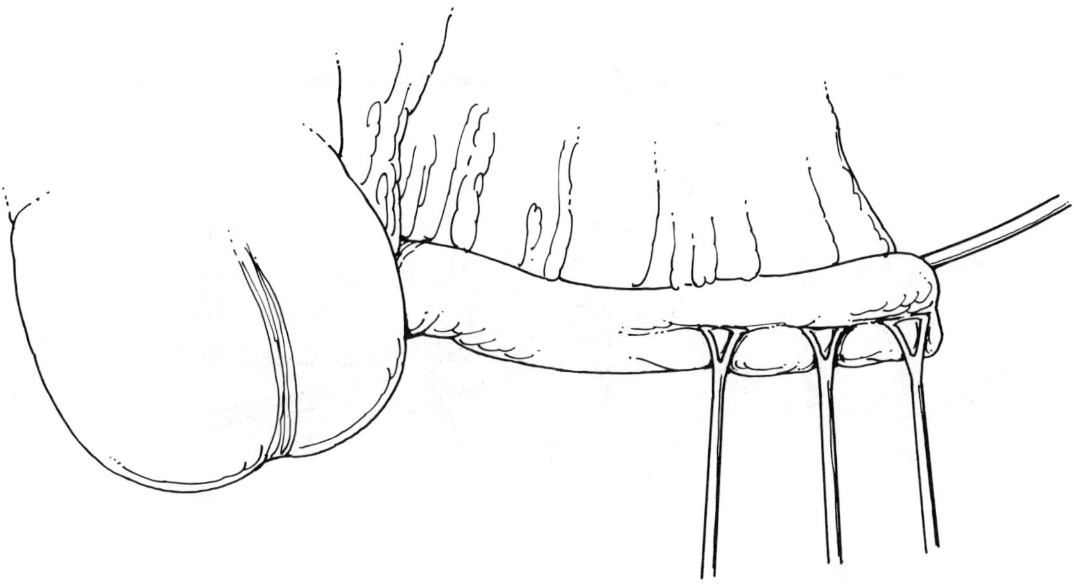

Figure 17-2A. A 12 French catheter is passed through the efferent limb and is positioned adjacent to the mesentery. Babcock clamps are used to grasp the antimesenteric surface of the terminal ileum.

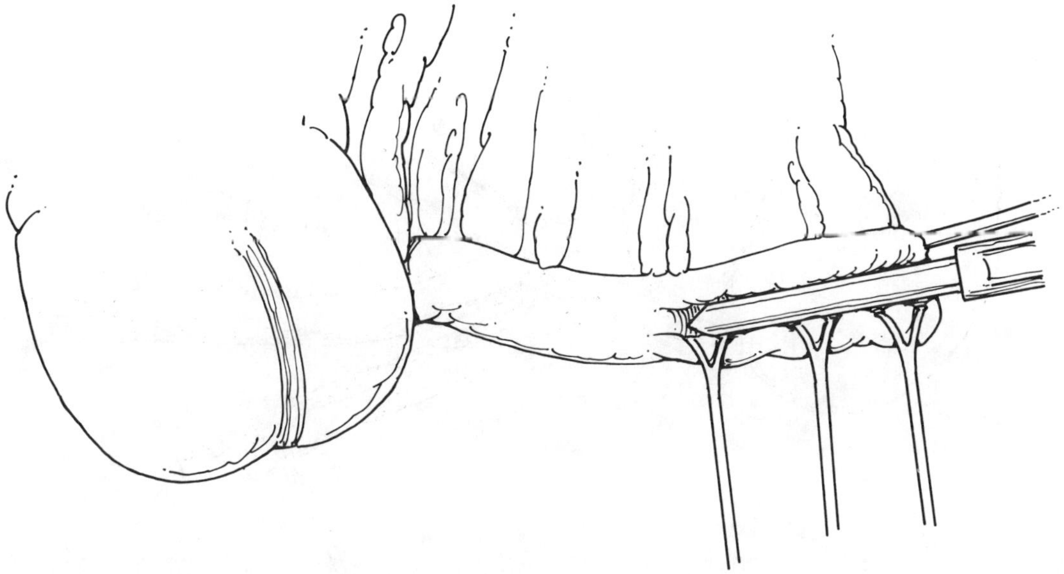

Figure 17-2B. A 6-cm GIA stapler is used to remove the redundant antimesenteric portion of the terminal ileum. Enough tissue should be removed to prevent sideways motion of the catheter; however, there should not be any tension on the bowel wall over the catheter. An 18 French catheter will be needed later for emptying the reservoir.

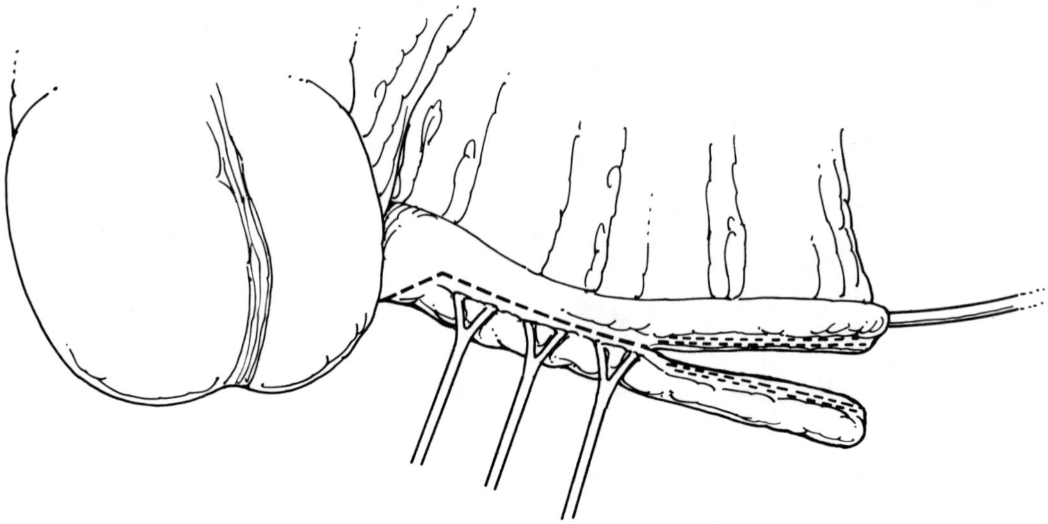

Figure 17-2C. Additional applications of the GIA stapler are made along the dashed lines.

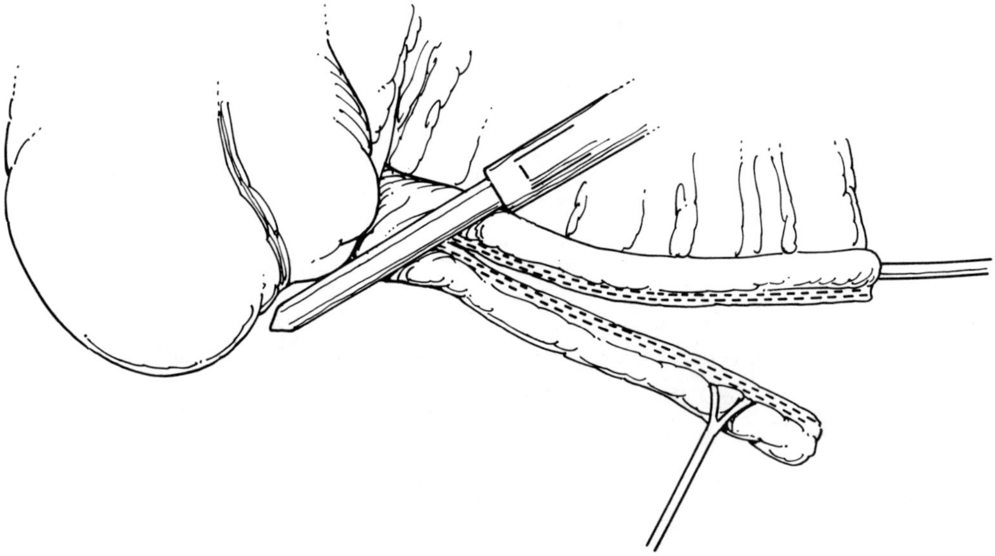

Figure 17-2D. The last application of the GIA stapler is made at an angle to avoid entry of the staple line into the cecum.

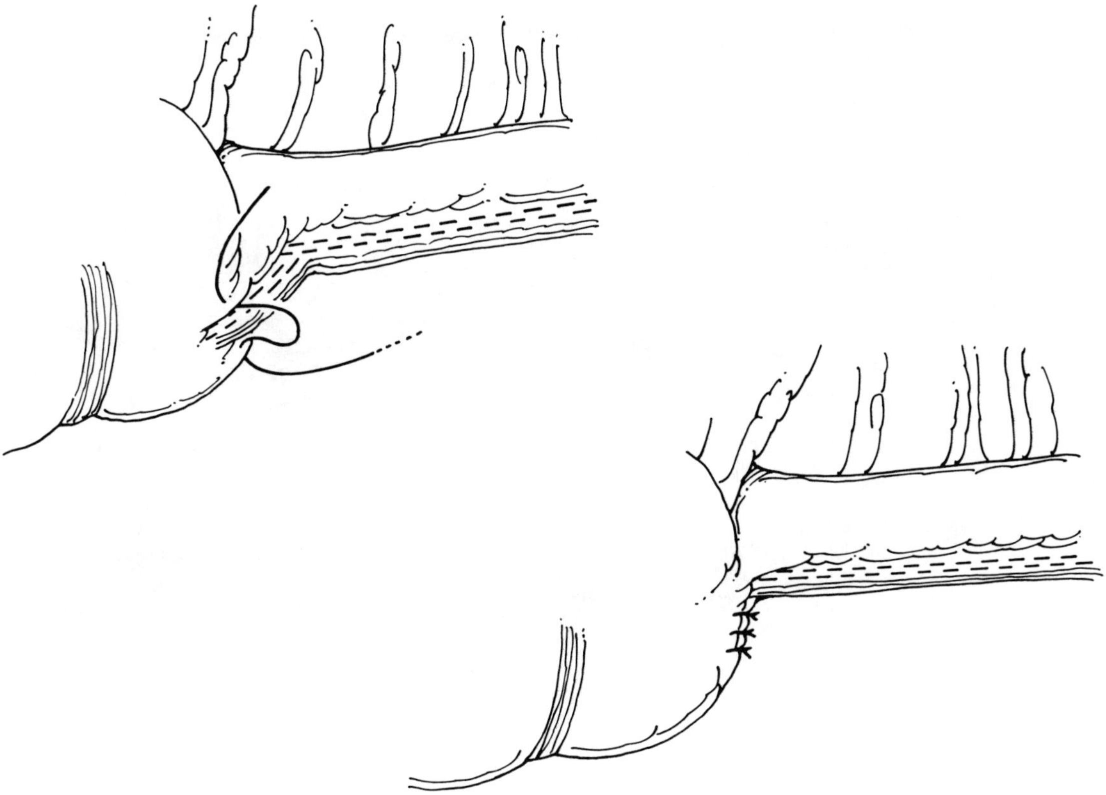

Figure 17-2E. As shown in the drawing at left, the resultant funnel-shaped ileocolic junction is plicated with 3-0 silk Lembert sutures to reinforce the ileocecal valve. After 5 or 6 Lembert plication sutures have been placed (drawing at right), the ileocecal valve should be noticeably narrowed. The funnel-shaped configuration is altered to a straight tube of efferent limb meeting the cecum at a right angle.

of the bladder or disruption of the ureters or bladder neck if performed low in the bladder. In my opinion, this procedure should be reserved for patients with medical contraindications to major open surgery.

Numerous institutions and cooperative groups are performing protocol studies of neoadjuvant and adjuvant chemotherapy in addition to cystectomy. Each of these approaches has its advantages and disadvantages. Although a similar approach has been used in testicular cancer, the protocol completion rates in bladder cancer are not nearly as high as in testis cancer. The main reason is that patients with bladder cancer on average are considerably older than testicular cancer patients.

In most patients undergoing radical cystectomy, a full bilateral pelvic lymph node dissection is performed. If the frozen sections are negative, then the radical cystec-

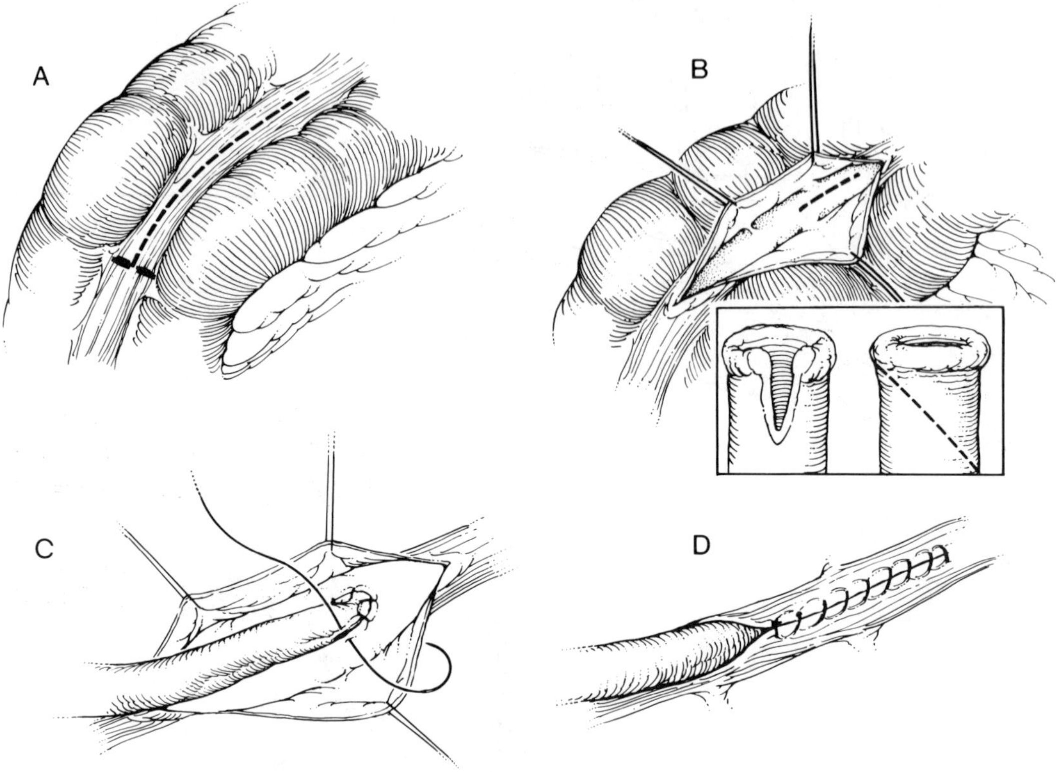

Figure 17-3. In drawing A, the sites for ureteral implantation along the tenia are selected to allow a smooth course of the ureter. A T-shaped incision is made in the tenia. The crossbar of the T will be at the hiatus of the ureteral implantation. This maneuver helps prevent obstruction of the ureter as it enters the hiatus of the tunnel. 17-3B—. A mucosal incision is made to create the orifice; the ureter is cut obliquely or spatulated to increase the size of the anastomosis. 17-3C—. About 6 sutures of 5-0 synthetic monofilament abosorbable suture are used for the anatomosis. 17-3D—. The tunnel is closed over the ureter with a 5-0 synthetic braided nonabsorbable suture. A running locked stitch is used to prevent shortening of the tunnel. The goal of the implantation is to provide a tunnel that is 4-5 times the diameter of the ureter in length.

tomy is carried out. If the nodes are grossly positive or if there are multiple microscopically positive nodes, the procedure is normally terminated. If the patient is having significant local symptoms of pain, frequency, or bleeding, usually an ileal conduit is created for palliation. The patient would then be considered for cytoreduction with chemotherapy.

If the lymph nodes are microscopically negative, a radical cystectomy is performed. Some centers apply a nerve-sparing technique to the cystectomy similar to that developed for a radical prostatectomy. The choice of urinary diversion encompasses an ileal or colon conduit, a continent urinary reservoir such as a Kock pouch, a Mainz pouch, or an Indian continent urinary reservoir; or a neobladder such as a modified Mainz or Hautmann procedure.

Urinary Diversions

Ileal conduits and colon conduits have been standard procedures for many years. The complication rates and reoperation rates are well established. The incidence of tumor in the isolated bowel segments is extremely low compared to the rate for those bowel segments in which both urine and feces are in contact with the mucosa.

Continent reservoirs offer the advantage of not requiring the patient to wear an ostomy appliance. However, for the procedure to be successful, patients must be highly motivated and willing to put forth a small amount of extra effort in terms of taking care of themselves and their continent reservoir. Patients need to have a degree of manual dexterity in order to perform intermittent catherization necessary to take care of a continent reservoir. They must also have normal or nearly normal bowel and renal function in order to have adequate reserves of these organ systems after a continent reservoir is provided. The risk of tumor formation in the bowel segments used for the reservoir in the postoperative period is unknown. These patients require careful follow-up. They are evaluated preoperatively to make certain that they do not have any polypoid lesions prior to diversion.

In the last couple of years, a great deal of enthusiasm has developed for the neobladder. Several similar procedures have evolved using colon and/or small bowel to create the neobladder. The reservoir is hooked up to the urethra and the patient voids by performing a Valsalva's maneuver if possible. Again, long-term follow-up will be required to make certain that there is not an increased incidence of tumors in the bowel segment or in the urethra.

Summary

The role of cystectomy in the management of bladder cancer will certainly continue to evolve. The number of patients requiring cystectomy may decline considerably if multimodal therapies are successful. Long-term follow-up of the different treatment strategies will be needed before any final decisions can be made about the role of surgery in the care of invasive bladder cancer.

18

CURRENT CONCEPTS FOR CHEMOTHERAPY IN ADVANCED AND EARLY UROTHELIAL TRACT NEOPLASMS

Alan Yagoda, M.D.

UROTHELIAL TRACT TUMORS (RENAL pelvis, ureter, urinary bladder, urethra, and prostatic ducts), which represent 4.7% (6.8% and 2.5% in men and women, respectively) of all malignancies in the United States annually, account for 49,000 cases and 10,400 (0.2%) deaths; they are the seventh leading cause of cancer-related death in men and fourteenth in women.

About 66-75% of cases present with local disease, whereas 13% have regional and 20% distant metastases. Most patient are seen initially with superficial noninvasive lesions (Cis, Ta, T1), which are treated successfully with complete response (CR) in 60% with intravesically administered bacille Calmette-Guérin (BCG). Of interest, recent data suggest that BCG induces interleukin-2. Other active intravesical agents—although less efficacious than BCG—are mitomycin-C (MIT), thiophosphoramide (thio-tepa) and Adriamycin (ADR). Recent trials have explored interferon, tumor necrosis factor and interleukin-2; none has yet been proven superior to BCG.

Chemical Agents for Advanced Disease

Efficacious single agents for advanced disease are cisplatin (DDP) (30% remission rate; 95% confidence interval [CI]=25-35%) and methotrexate (MTX) (30%; CI=25-35%), as well as vinblastine (VLB) (16%; CI=8-24%) and ADR (17%; CI=12-22%).[1] Others demonstrating some antitumor activity are amsacrine, 5-fluorouracil (5-FU), and hexamethylmelamine (HMM), the last being active for bilharzial bladder cancer.

Many multidrug combinations have been tried, but the most frequently employed include DDP + ADR (CA regimen) with or without cyclophosphamide (CTX) (CAP or CISCA), and DDP + MTX (MP) together or with VLB (CMV or MCV) and ADR (M-VAC). Complete and partial (PR) remissions have been described in CI=43-69% of patients given CA and CI=41-51% with CISCA; in limited randomized trials, the superiority of these regimens has been difficult to prove. MP regimens have been evaluated in low and high dosages, as well as in various schedules in order to avoid nephrotoxicity. Although response occurs in CI=41-53% of cases, a randomized trial comparing MP to DDP alone found no statistical difference for response (45% and 33%, respectively) or survival (8.7 and 7.2 mo, respectively). Although 26% CR + 16% PR are noted in 62 CMV cases and CI=48-66% in 115 from published phase 2 trials, overall median survival is identical (7-8 mo) to that reported for MP.

In contrast, M-VAC[2] is superior for response and survival ($p < 0.0001$) when compared to DDP and to CISCA in phase 3 prospective randomized trials in >350 cases.[3,4] The standard M-VAC dosage schedule is 30 mg/m^2 of MTX on day 1 followed by 30 mg/m^2 of ADR + 3 mg/m^2 of VLB + 70 mg/m^2 of DDP on day 2, with MTX + VLB given together on days 15 and 21. Cycles are repeated q.28-35 days, depending on mucositis, renal function, and myelosuppression. Overall median survival for M-VAC was 12.5 versus 8.3 mo for cisplatin,[3] and 82 versus 40 wk for CISCA.[4] Metastatic sites responding included lung, bone, intra-abdominal, and primary lesions—particularly those with N+ disease; least responsive were liver lesions and nontransitional cell histologies. A more intense—and apparently effective—M-VAC dose (ADR doubled to 60 mg/m^2 and VLB to 4 mg/m^2 and DDP to 100 mg/m^2) was possible with the addition of GM-CSF, which produced a 40% remission rate in 32 M-VAC/CISCA progressors.[5] Prospective trials are evaluating GM-CSF + M-VAC given q.3 wk.

Neoadjuvant Phase 2 Studies

Many neoadjuvant phase 2 studies have reported clinical tumor downstaging in the bladder primary in 50->60% of cases, with CR in >25-35%; however, the clinical versus pathological staging error following cystectomy is >30-50%, and the true (pathologically-proven) CR rate is closer to 22-30%.[6] In addition, any improvement in survival following neoadjuvant chemotherapy not infrequently is due to the number of small (T2) conceivably low-grade or papillary cancers included in the series, a group of tumors that have a relatively good 5-yr survival rate. Although bladder preservation can be attained in selected cases, most patients remain at risk for the development of de novo tumors. Of more importance, perhaps, is the finding that patients whose tumors are downstaged to PO, Pis, Pa, and Pl survive longer than those who fail neoadjuvant therapy; in fact, progressors who go on to standard therapy will die more rapidly than reported. Such data indicate that DDP-based neoadjuvant therapy separates "good-risk" from "poor-risk" groups. For example, in 56 responders, 90% were surviving >3 years, versus only 25% of 67 progressors.[7] However, only randomized phase 3 studies will determine benefit.

References

1. Yagoda A. The role of cisplatin-based chemotherapy in advanced urothelial tract cancer. Semin Oncol 1989; 16 (suppl 6):98-104.
2. Sternberg C, Yagoda A, Scher HI, et al. Methotrexate, vinblastine, doxorubicin, and cisplatin for transitional cell carcinoma of the urothelium:efficacy and patterns of response and relapse. Cancer 1989; 64:2448-58.
3. Loehrer PJ, Elson P, Kuebler JP, et al. Advanced bladder cancer:a prospective intergroup trial comparing single-agent cisplatin (CDDP) versus M-VAC combination therapy. Proc Amer Soc Clin Oncol 1990; 9(abstract 511):132.
4. Logothetis CJ, Dexeus FH, Finn L, et al. A prospective randomized trial comparing M-VAC and CISCA chemotherapy for patients with metastatic urothelial tumors. J Clin Oncol 1990; 8:1050-62.
5. Logothetis CJ, Dexeus F, Sella A, et al. Escalated therapy for refractory urothelial tumors:methotrexate-vinblastine-doxorubicin-cisplatin plus unglycosylated recombinant human granulocyte-macrophage colony-stimulating factor. JNCI 1990; 82:667-72.
6. Scher H, Herr H, Sternberg C, et al. Neoadjuvant chemotherapy for invasive bladder cancer:experience with the M-VAC regimen. Brit J Urol 1989; 64:250-56.
7. Splinter TAW, Denis L, Scher H, et al. Neoadjuvant chemotherapy of urinary bladder cancer:the prognostic value of local tumor response. In:Murphy GP, Khoury D, eds. Int Symp on Ther Prog in Urol Cancers. New York:AR Liss, 1989; 557-62.

19

ROLE OF PRIMARY RETROPERITONEAL LYMPH NODE DISSECTION IN CLINICAL STAGE A NONSEMINOMATOUS GERM CELL TESTIS CANCER

J. P. Donohue, M.D.; J. A. Thornhill, M.Ch., F.R.C.S.I.;
R. S. Foster, M.D.; R. G. Rowland, M.D.; and R. Bihrle, M.D.

Introduction

ALMOST 1,200 NONSEMINOMATOUS GERM cell (NSGC) testis cancer patients underwent retroperitoneal lymph node dissection (RPLND) at Indiana University Medical Center (IUMC) in the period 1965-89. This represents the largest institutional series of surgical testis cancer cases, and it is therefore timely to review our results for each stage of disease. This paper deals with a subgroup of patients who underwent primary RPLND (n=638)—specifically those who were considered clinically to have stage A disease before surgery (n=464, no demonstrable metastases by clinical, radiological, and serological methods).

Options for managing clinical stage A NSGC testis cancer after orchiectomy include the surgical approach involving primary RPLND.[1] Alternatively, nonsurgical treatment options include routine abdominal irradiation or selective combination chemotherapy.[2] The most conservative approach involves surveillance or a "wait and see" policy after orchiectomy.[3] With this last approach, chemotherapy is reserved for patients who subsequently relapse.

The choice of management in clinical stage A disease is one of the most controversial topics in urological oncology today. Interestingly, the dichotomy of views between the surgical versus the conservative approach has geographic trends influenced

The authors thank Jonathan Messemer for his help in systems analysis. J. Thornhill was supported by the Irish Cancer Society.

by the various medical specialities that have historically managed these cases in different countries. In the United States, with its strong urologic surgical tradition, primary RPLND has been consistently advocated since this operation was popularized in the 1920s.[4] In contrast, in the United Kingdom the conservative approach is generally favored. Routine abdominal irradiation was standard treatment there[5,6] until surveillance was introduced in 1979 as an alternate method.[7] Unfortunately, this controversy about the optimal choice of management has been exacerbated by a lack of comparative data. It has not been possible to compare the results of conservative management, which are based on clinical staging methods, with surgical data based on more accurate surgical pathological staging. This study is the first in the literature to analyze the results of primary RPLND based on prior *clinical* staging of patients. It was specifically designed so that surgical results over a 25-year period would be directly comparable with those using the conservative approach.

Patients and Methods

Between 1965 and 1989, 464 patients with clinical stage A NSGC testis cancer underwent primary RPLND at IUMC. Clinical stage A disease was defined as no radiological evidence of metastatic disease, and the serum tumor markers alpha-fetoprotein (AFP) and beta human choriogonadotropin (HCG) were either normal or diminished according to their known half-life after orchiectomy. Average age of patients was 28 yr (median: 27 yr; range: 1-53 yr). One patient had a past history of testis cancer (stage A seminoma in the contralateral testis treated by orchiectomy and prophylactic abdominal irradiation), and 3% of patients (n=15) had a family history for testis cancer.

The site of the primary tumor was the right testis in 55% and the left in 44% of cases; 1 case had bilateral synchronous tumors. Of the total, 6% of cases (n=27) had a history of cryptorchidism, including ipsilateral or bilateral maldescent with orchiopexy (3.5%, n=16); maldescent without prior correction (1.3%, n=6); and contralateral cryptorchidism (1.1%, n=5). A total of 58% of patients were married or divorced, of whom 54% had fathered children.

The average duration of symptoms was 2.5 mo (median: 1.2 mo: range: 0 - 35 mo). Of the 16% of patients (n=75) who had diagnostic scrotal ultrasound, 91% of scans supported the diagnosis; the remainder were equivocal or normal. Nearly all (98%) patients had their orchiectomy at outside hospitals; 37 cases (8%) had scrotal violation at the time of orchiectomy (2 had hemiscrotectomy before referral).

Clinical staging after orchiectomy included abdominal CT scan in 84% of patients; the rest had lymphangiography, ultrasound, or IVP, depending on the year of presentation. Chest CT scan or whole-lung tomograms were routinely performed. AFP and beta HCG were assayed in 90% of patients from 1979 onward. Five patients with normal radiology but persistently raised serum markers were excluded from analyses.

Four surgeons performed 99% of RPLND operations, including 61% by one surgeon (J.P.D.). Modifications in surgical technique during this period included a downscaling of the resection template based on improved knowledge of the sites of nodal metastases.[8] Nerve-sparing techniques were also introduced in order to preserve ejaculatory function.[9] Fifty-four patients (12%) had a full bilateral RPLND below the level of the renal vessels. Another 170 patients (37%) had an extended suprahilar dissection, and 240 patients (52%) had a modified unilateral RPLND. More than one-third (36%) of patients (n=167) had prospective nerve-sparing during RPLND, the majority of whom had a modified unilateral lymph node dissection. A midline transperitoneal approach was routinely used (99%) and only 3 cases had a thoracoabdominal incision. Additional procedures during RPLND included nephrectomy (n=2), en bloc caval resection with tumor (n=1), hemiscrotectomy (n=26), appendectomy (n=79), and testis prosthesis (n=3).

For analyses, patients were divided in 2 groups, depending on their year of surgery—1965-78 (n=86) and 1979-89 (n=378). This categorization was chosen for several reasons: Surveillance was introduced in 1979 as an alternative to surgery; from 1979 onward, clinical staging became more elaborate, and 90% of cases had CT scans and serum marker assays; and effective combination platinum chemotherapy was generally available from 1979.

All cases histories of patients undergoing RPLND at IUMC since 1965 are fully computerized. The duration of follow-up is wide ranging (0.2 - 276 mo). Mean follow-up varies from 99 mo for cases treated before 1979 to 30 mo for those treated from 1979 onward.

Results

Between 1965 and 1978, 86 patients with clinical stage A disease underwent primary RPLND (results are shown in table 19-1). Surgical pathological staging confirmed that 66% of cases (n=57) were truly pathological stage A, but the remaining 34%

Table 19-1. Primary RPLND in Clinical Stage A NSGC Testis Cancer: Results, 1965-1978

Disease extent (path. stage)	No. patients/ (%)	No. relapses/ (%)	Survival (%)	No. deaths
Path. stage A	57 (66)	6 (11)	100	0
Path. stage B No adjuvant	9 (11)	4 (44)	100	0
Path. stage B Plus adjuvant*	20 (23)	3 (15)	95	1**
All cases	86	13 (15)	98.8	1

* Nonplatinum-based chemotherapy ± abdominal irradiation
** 1 death from testis cancer

(n=29) had cancerous nodes removed at RPLND. Nearly one fifth (18%) of patients (n=15) had pathological stage B1 disease (retroperitoneal nodes <2.5 cm in diameter and/or <5 nodes involved), and 16% of cases (n=14) had pathological stage B2 disease (2.5 - 10 cm diameter or >5 nodes). These figures highlight the inaccuracy of clinical staging during this period.

The relapse rate for pathological stage A patients was 11% (n=6). All relapses were pulmonary and went into remission following single- or double-agent cytotoxics (n=6) and further surgery (n=1); no cancer deaths were seen in this subgroup. The relapse rate among 29 patients with pathological stage B disease was 24% (n=7). Nine patients had not received postoperative adjuvant therapy, of whom 4 relapsed (44%). Twenty patients had received some form of postoperative adjuvant treatment (variable regimes including dactinomycin and/or irradiation), among whom the relapse rate was 15% (n=3). Relapse occurred in the lungs (n=5), lungs plus mediastinum (n=1), and pelvis (n=1); another case had marker elevation only. Salvage treatment included various nonplatinum cytotoxic regimens (n=4) combined with further surgery (n=1), surgery alone (n=2), or combined with irradiation (XRT) (n=1). One death from disseminated disease occurred at 2 yr, but this was the only cancer death among all 86 patients undergoing primary RPLND 1965-79.

Table 19-2 shows a comparison of these early surgical results with equivalent data using routine abdominal XRT for clinical stage A disease. The overall relapse of 15% after RPLND equates with the 17% relapse after prophylactic XRT.[10] However, the long-term survival of 98.8% after RPLND surpasses that after XRT, where 14 - 18% of cases ultimately died of disease.[11,3]

Findings in Surgical Staging

The majority of patients in this series underwent RPLND between 1979 and 1989 (n=378, table 19-3). Surgical staging confirmed that 71% of clinical stage A patients (n=267) had pathological stage A disease, while 29% of patients (n=111) had positive nodes at operation (stage B1 = 25% [n=93] and stage B2 = 5% [n=18]). These figures again illustrate the unsatisfactory false-negative staging error using currently available clinical staging methods.

Table 19-2. Comparison of Results in Clinical Stage A NSGC Testis Cancer Using Abdominal Irradiation or Primary RPLND

Primary treatment	Period	No. patients	Relapse (%)	Survival (%)
Abdominal irradiation[1,2]	1962-79	147	17	87
RPLND[3]	1965-79	86	15	98.8

[1,2] Derived from Tyrrell and Peckham (1976) and Peckham (1982)

[3] Present series, Indiana University Medical Center

Table 19-3. Primary RPLND in Clinical Stage A NSGC Testis Cancer: Results, 1979-89

Disease extent (path. stage)	No. patients/ (%)	No. relapses/ (%)	Survival (%)	No. deaths
Path. stage A	267 (71)	29 (11)	99.2	2*
Path. stage B No adjuvant	65 (17)	21 (32)	98.5	1**
Path. stage B Plus adjuvant	46 (12)	0 (0)	100	0
All cases	378	50 (13)	99.2	3

* 2 deaths (1 cancer, 1 postoperative)
** 1 cancer death

The relapse rate among pathological stage A patients (11%, n=29) was consistent with the earlier time period. Sites of relapse included lungs (n=14), mediastinum (n=5), lungs plus mediastinum (n=1), lungs plus liver (n=1), pelvis (n=2), liver (n=1), and groin (n=2); 3 patients had serum marker elevation alone. Treatment at relapse involved combination platinum chemotherapy in 28 patients, with further operative intervention in 6 of these; 1 patient underwent surgical resection alone. Two patients died in this pathological stage A subgroup. One patient died 8 days postoperatively from fulminant sepsis, relating to a urinary tract infection and a cardiac septal defect, which became manifest during fluid resuscitation as acute respiratory distress syndrome. The other death was a relapsing patient who died of disseminated disease despite salvage treatment.

The relapse rate among patients with pathological stage B disease (n=111) was 19% (n=21). Sites included lungs (n=10), mediastinum (n=1), pelvis (n=1), and liver plus retroperitoneum (n=1); 2 patients had disseminated disease and another 6 relapsed with marker elevation only. The decision whether or not to give post-RPLND adjuvant chemotherapy (2 courses of platinum in combination) in pathological stage B cases was governed by a randomized clinical trial in operation during most of this period.[12] None of the 46 patients who received adjuvant chemotheraphy suffered relapse. In contrast, 32% (n=21) of the 65 patients who had no adjuvant chemotherapy went on to relapse; in stage B1 (n=54), the relapse rate was 31% (n=17); in stage B2 disease (n=11), the relapse rate was 36% (n=4). Relapse was treated by combination chemotherapy (n=20) with subsequent surgery (n=4) or XRT (n=1); 1 patient had surgical resection alone. There was 1 cancer death in this pathological stage B group; overall, 3 patients died (2 from cancer and 1 postoperatively) among 378 patients treated 1979-89.

Table 19-4 compares the surgical results (1979-89) with contemporary series using surveillance in prestigious centers around the world. The relapse rate with surveillance is 25-35%.[13,14] This is higher than the 13% in this surgical series. Consequently, the mortality rate from cancer (or related to treatment) is also less in the surgical group (n=3, 0.8%) than in surveillance series (0.9 - 4.4% of cases).[14,15]

Table 19-4. Primary RPLND versus Surveillance in Clinical Stage A NSGC Testis Cancer

Investigator	No. patients	Relapses (%)	Survival (%)	No. deaths
Primary RPLND				
Donohue	378	13	99.2	3
Surrveillance				
Freedman	259	32	98.8	3
Raghavan	46	28	95.6	2
Thompson	36	33	97.2	1
Liedke	107	35	99.1	2
Sogani	102	25	97.1	3

Table 19-5. Primary RPLND in Clinical Stage A NSGC Testis Cancer, 1965-89

Disease extent (path. stage)	No. patients/ (%)	No. relapses/ (%)	Survival (%)	No. deaths
Path. stage A	324 (70)	35 (11)	99.1	2*
Path. stage B No adjuvant	74 (16)	25 (34)	98.6	1**
Path. stage B Plus adjuvant	66 (14)	3 (4)	98.5	1
All cases	464	63 (14)	99.1	4

* 1 cancer, 1 postoperative death
** 2 cancer deaths

Results Over 25 Years

The combined results using primary RPLND over 25 yr (1965-89) are shown in table 19-5. The preoperative false-negative staging error of 30% using clinical methods was consistent throughout this period. The relapse rate of 11% in pathological stage A patients and 34% in pathological stage B patients not given adjuvant chemotherapy also showed little variation during this extended time frame. However, the relapse rate of 4% in pathological stage B patients who were given postoperative adjuvant treatment reflects a combination of cases treated, both in the preplatinum era (relapse = 15%) and when effective combination chemotherapy became widely available (relapse = 0%). Overall, only 4 out of 464 patients treated by primary RPLND died of cancer (n=3) or treatment-related causes (n=1). Another 2 patients subsequently died of proven unrelated conditions.

Discussion

The dual aim of the management of NSGC testis cancer is to minimize disease relapse and to optimize survival. This basic principle is as pertinent today as it was in the past, for despite major advancements in diagnostic radiology, immunology, and chemotherapy during recent decades, NSGC testis cancer remains a most rapidly growing and potentially lethal tumor. The reasons for performing primary RPLND in clinical stage A disease are to achieve absolute precision in disease staging and to take therapeutic action if resected nodes are positive. The magnitude of this series provides a unique opportunity to statistically analyze and critically appraise our surgical result. Also, the time span of the study—covering 2 different medical eras—allows us to better define the current role for primary RPLND.

The purpose of reporting our early results (1965-78) was to provide a direct comparison between primary RPLND and primary abdominal radiation in clinical stage A disease that was not previously available. The results confirmed a 34% false-negative staging error in this early period using clincial methods alone. This was not unexpected, because the inaccuracy of clinical examination, IVU, and lymphangiography are known. It was not until the advent of second generation CT technology and serum tumor markers that clinical staging achieved a more acceptable—albeit limited—level of sophistication.[16] Accurate surgical staging was an important prognostic indicator for individual patients by defining those most at risk of relapse. Unfortunately, however, this diagnostic accuracy could not be used to full advantage because there was not truly effective adjuvant treatment available at that time.

Therapeutic Benefit of RPLND

The obvious merit of RPLND was its therapeutic benefit if nodes were positive; 68% of all pathological stage B cases were cured by RPLND alone. The other feature of RPLND was that it conferred a clear advantage on patients who did subsequently relapse. Such patients proved to be curable, in marked contrast to those relapsing in series using abdominal XRT.[10,11] The reason for this was two-fold:

1. RPLND cleared the retroperitoneum as a site of relapse; subsequent deposits occurred in the lungs alone and were easily detected by simple radiographic methods. This was not the case in XRT series, where retroperitoneal relapse was not difficult to detect.

2. The disease model of lung deposits alone (in 15% of cases after RPLND) was curable even with the limited cytotoxic drugs available.

Only 1 of 13 relapsers died of cancer, whereas all relapsing cases (14-18%) in XRT series died of disease. This significant survival advantage with RPLND over XRT favors surgery as the most appropriate approach in clinical stage A disease during this early period. We believe that the same analogy will apply in the future, when "high-risk" clinical stage A disease will be treated with systemic chemotherapy. Some will fail and recur in the retroperitoneum, and the relapse pattern will be attenuated over time, especially those with teratocarcinoma and teratomatous elements in their primary testis tumors.

Ongoing Referral Signifies Broad Support

Between 1979 and 1989, more patients were treated surgically in this series than in any reported series using the surveillance approach. This ongoing referral of patients for surgery from oncologists and urologists throughout the United States signifies broad support for this management approach. The results show that clinical staging remained inaccurate during the current time period despite routine CT and serum marker evaluation. The false-negative clinical staging error rate of 29% is not acceptable as a basis for defining further treatment requirements. The inaccuracy of CT is due to its inability to detect derangements in internal nodal architecture, especially if nodes are of normal size.[17] This is particularly relevant because 84% of patients with surgical pathological stage B disease were designated as stage B1 (<5 nodes involved). Frequently, these cases had microscopic disease.

The relapse rate in pathological stage A cases remained consistent with our earlier results (11%). It is reassuring that downscaling the operative resection template did not cause any increase in relapse. Relapse occurred outside the operative field; therefore, RPLND achieved its technical aim. However, this relapsing group of 11% are of concern, especially because 1 patient (out of 267) ultimately died of cancer. A retrospective analysis of pathological stage A cases is needed to identify a specific high-risk subgroup with a view to more intensive postoperative follow-up. As in other similar studies, this would concentrate principally on histopathology of the primary testis tumor.[18]

The major therapeutic benefit of RPLND was clearly evident in pathological stage B cases. Results in those cases in which postoperative adjuvant chemotherapy was given (n=65) confirm that 68% of all stage B cases (B1 and B2) are cured by surgery alone. Moreover, these cases have already proven their metastatic potential. However satisfactory these results, the relapse rate of 32% after RPLND alone contrasted with the 0% relapse and 100% survival among those who received adjuvant chemotherapy. These findings support but do not mandate a 2-cycle postoperative regimen of a platinum combination. The ease of follow-up for both patient and physician in this setting would outweigh the short-term toxicity of adjuvant chemotherapy. The only pathological stage B patient in this series who died of cancer had not received any postoperative adjuvant treatment. Other authors who advocate the withholding of adjuvant chemotherapy generally limit this approach to stage B1 disease.[19] Their reasoning is that relapse is less in stage B1 than in stage B2 disease. However, in this series the relapse rate was not significantly reduced among the 2 groups (31% and 36%, respectively). These results would tend to support the use of adjuvant chemotherapy even in limited stage B1 disease.

Pros and Cons of Surveillance

Advocates of surveillance base their approach on the hypothesis that any patients who relapse after orchiectomy can be salvaged by chemotherapy when metastases become manifest. The aim is laudable, in that most cases should require no further treatment other than orchiectomy, and the toxicity of treatment is acceptable in the minority who subsequently require chemotherapy. Although initial reports of a 15% relapse rate and no deaths were a strong impetus to adopting this approach, these results unfortunately were both premature and misleading.[20,21] Most subsequent series (already quoted) show that the relapse rate is about double that originally reported, and relapse increases with each year of follow-up.[22]

The difficulty in detecting early retroperitoneal relapse is now also recognized, and reports emphasizing the importance of back pain in diagnosis serve to highlight the inaccuracy of current clinical investigative methods.[23] The most serious drawback of surveillance, however, is not its increasingly obvious high relapse rate but the associated death rate among patients who relapse. In all reports previously cited, 10% of relapsing patients die of testis cancer. Even some of the strongest protagonists of surveillance now admit that the ideal protocol has yet to be developed.[15] In contrast, in this 1979-89 series, only 3 of 378 patients died.

These surgical results spanning 25 yr are therefore unmatched by any conservative approach over the same timespan. The rationale for primary RPLND was clearly vindicated and deserves reiteration; there is absolute precision in disease staging, and subsequent treatment requirements can be clearly defined. There is undoubted therapeutic benefit if nodes are positive. There is considerable ease of follow-up, for patient and clinician alike. Finally, the disease model is altered in the event of relapse. Relapse does not occur in the retroperitoneum; rather, it occurs in the lungs, making it easier to detect and easier to treat than the disease model of retroperitoneum-plus-lungs as seen with surveillance.

Theoretically, surveillance is an attractive alternative to RPLND because it spares routine abdominal operation after orchiectomy. Also, the approach has provided valuable insight into the natural history of testis cancer. In practice, however, we would have difficulty in accepting the increased risk of relapse and the subsequent loss of about 10% of relapsing patients in order to spare patients a straightforward operative procedure. This controversy between surveillance and primary RPLND would largely disappear if a reliable method of detecting micrometastasis were developed. However, until that time, these comprehensive results strongly support a valid role for primary RPLND (as perhaps the more appropriate approach) in clinical stage A nonseminomatous germ cell testis tumors.

The entire question of primary RPLND versus surveillance should be reopened in communities committed to a single nonsurgical approach in clinical stage A disease. We do not urge that surveillance should be suddenly abandoned, as this clearly will not happen. Rather, medical oncologists should be fully aware that primary nerve-sparing RPLND is at least competitive and indeed marginally superior to surveillance in many respects. In the light of these findings and with continuing study of risk/benefit and cost analysis, we may soon realize that the patient is better served by having an informed choice of either conservative or surgical management options in low clinical stage NSGCT.

Summary

Results with primary RPLND in 464 patients with clinical stage A NSGC testis cancer treated over 25 years (1965-89) were reviewed. Results were subdivided into early (1965-78) and contemporary (1979-89) in order to be directly comparable with series using XRT or surveillance. Between 1965 and 1978 (86 clincical stage A patients), the overall relapse of 15% (n=13) was similar to that with XRT series, but survival (98.8% after RPLND) was superior to that achieved with irradiation (87%). From 1979 to 1989, 378 clinical stage A cases had primary RPLND, of whom 29% (n=111) had cancerous nodes. The relapse rate for pathological stage A cases (n=267) was 11%; 2 patients died. The relapse in pathological stage B cases without adjuvant chemotherapy was 32%. No relapse was seen among 46 pathological stage B cases given postoperative adjuvant chemotherapy. The overall relapse rate of 13% in clinical stage A cases is less than the 30% rate seen with surveillance. Also, there were only 3 deaths among 378 RPLND cases, whereas almost 10% of all relapsers in collected surveillance series died of testis cancer. These consistent results using RPLND over 25 yr suggest a survival advantage in eliminating the retroperitoneum as a site of relapse. Now that morbidity of RPLND is essentially eliminated, primary RPLND is supported as a most appropriate treatment for clinical stage A disease.

References

1. Donohue JP. Selecting initial therapy seminoma and nonseminoma. Cancer 1987; 60(3):115-20.
2. Pont J, Holtl W, Kosak D, et al. Risk adapted treatment choice in stage I nonseminomatous testicular germ cell cancer by regarding vascular invasion in the primary tumor: a prospective trial. J Clin Oncol 1990; 8(1):16-20.
3. Peckham MJ. Radiotherapy for clinical stage I and II nonseminomatous germ cell tumours (malignant teratoma) of the testis. In: Williams CJ, Whitehouse JMA, eds. Recent advances in clinical oncology. Edinburgh, London, Melbourne, New York: Churchill Livingstone, 1982.
4. Hinman F. The radical operation for teratoma testis. Surg Syn Obstet 1919; 28:495-508.
5. Boden G, Gibb R. Radiotherapy and testicular neoplasms. Lancet 1951; 2:1195-97.
6. Peckham MJ, McElwain TJ. Radiotherapy of testicular tumours. Proc Roy Soc Med 1974; 67:300-03.
7. Peckham MJ, Barrett A, Husband JE, et al. Orchiectomy alone in testicular stage I nonseminomatous germ cell tumours. Lancet 1982; 2:678-80.
8. Donohue JP. Metastatic pathways of nonseminomatous germ cell cancers. Semin Urol 1984; 2:217-29.
9. Donohue JP, Thornhill JA, Foster RS, et al. The evolution of surgical templates and nerve-sparing techniques in retroperitoneal lymphadenectomy for low stage testis cancer. J Urol 1990; 143(4): 395A.
10. Tyrrell CJ, Peckham MJ. The response of lymph node metastases of testicular teratoma to radiation therapy. Brit J Urol 1976; 48:363-70.

11. Clements JC, McLeod DG, Weisbaum GS, et al. Radiation therapy for nonseminomatous germ cell tumour of the testis: a reappraisal. J Urol 1981; 126:490-92.
12. Williams SD, Stablein DM, Einhorn LH, et al. Immediate adjuvant chemotherapy versus observation with treatment at relapse in pathological stage II testicular cancer. N Engl J Med 1987; 317:1433-38.
13. Sogani PC, Fair WR. Surveillance alone in the treatment of clinical stage I nonseminomatous germ cell tumour of the testis (NSGCT). Semin Urol 1988; 6(1):53-56.
14. Liedke S, Allhoff EP, Jones U. Wait and see in NSGCT clinical stage I: a critical assessment after eight years. J Urol 1990; 143(4):397A.
15. Raghavan D, Colls B, Leir J, et al. Surveillance for stage I nonseminomatous germ cell tumours of the testis: the optimal protocol has not yet been developed. Br J Urol 1988; 61:522-26.
16. Rowland RG, Weisman D, Williams SD, et al. Accuracy of preoperative staging in stages A and B nonseminomatous germ cell testis tumours. J Urol 1982; 127:718-20.
17. Husband JE, MacDonald JS, Peckham MJ. Computed tomography in testicular disease: a review. J Roy Soc Med 1981; 74:441-47.
18. Young CF, Kalish LA, Brodsky GL, et al. Stage I nonseminomatous germ cell testis tumours; prediction of metastatic potential by primary histopathology. J Clin Oncol 1988; 6(9):1467-73.
19. Ritchie JP. Is adjuvant chemotherapy necessary for patients with stage B1 testicular cancer? J Urol 1990; 143(4):395A.
20. Read G, Johnson RJ, Wilkinson PM, et al. Prospective study of follow-up alone in stage I teratoma of the testis. Br Med J 1983; 287:1503-05.
21. Oliver RTD, Hope-Stone HF, Blandy JP. Justification of the use of surveillance in the management of stage I germ cell tumours of the testis. Br J Urol 1983; 55:760-63.
22. Freedman LS, Jones WG, Peckham MJ, et al. Histopathology in the prediction of relapse of patients with stage I testicular teratoma treated by orchiectomy alone. Lancet 1987; 2:294-98.
23. Smith DB, Newlands ES, Rustin GJS, et al. Lumbar pain in stage I testicular germ cell tumours: a symptom preceding radiological abnormality. Br J Urol 1989; 64:302-04.

20

WILMS' TUMOR

John Raffensperger, M.D.

WILMS' TUMOR, OR NEPHROBLASTOMA, is 1 of the 2 most common intra-abdominal tumors in childhood, occurring in 1 of 13,500 live births. It was one of the first tumors to respond to chemotherapy. As a result, the cure rate has improved from about 30% in 1960 to nearly 95% in 1990. For many years, almost all renal tumors in childhood were lumped together as "Wilms'" tumors, named after the German surgeon who published an extensive monograph on kidney tumors in 1899. At this time, a more precise diagnosis is required in order to arrive at optimum treatment of individual patients.

The typical tumor has a triphasic microscopic appearance consisting of epithelial and blastema cells with a connective tissue stroma. The epithelial cells may resemble renal tubules, which are interspersed with sheets of dark-staining blastema cells. The stroma may include any type of connective tissue, including smooth muscle, osteoid, or cartilage. In the late 1970s, 3 types of renal tumors were recognized as carrying a much more unfavorable prognosis. These included an anaplastic form, a rhabdoid tumor, and a clear-cell sarcoma. These 3 cell types account for only 10% of pediatric renal tumors, but account for nearly 60% of deaths. On the other hand, more benign forms of pediatric renal tumors have been identified. These include cystic nephroma, congenital mesoblastic nephroma, and nephroblastomatosis.

Classic Wilms' tumors distort the calyces and pelvis of the kidney and don't usually invade the renal capsule or metastasize until they are quite large. Metastases occur to regional lymph nodes and to the lung. Tumor may invade the renal vein and extend up the inferior vena cava to the right atrium. Liver metastases are rare, but tumors with unfavorable histology may metastasize to bone or to the brain.

There has long been a suspicion that Wilms' tumors have a genetic origin, since they are truly in the borderland between embryology and pathology. This was based upon the observed association of Wilms' tumors with birth defects such as aniridia, Beckwith syndrome, hemihypertrophy and genitourinary anomalies. Recent studies have identified deletion in the p13 region of chromosome 11 with syndromes associated with Wilms' tumors.

Clinically, children with Wilms' tumors are surprisingly asymptomatic until either a parent or a physician palpates an abdominal mass. Almost any imaging study, such as an intravenous pyelogram, abdominal ultrasound, or a CT scan, will demonstrate a tumor. Ultrasound provides additional information about the presence of tumor within the inferior vena cava or right atrium.

The treatment of Wilms' tumors, guided by several national cooperative study groups, has evolved from surgical excision combined with radiation and chemotherapy for all tumors to specific combinations of treatment that are defined by staging of the disease and the tumor's histology.

There continues to be controversy surrounding the optimum management of bilateral Wilms' tumors. Our preference is for primary bilateral "tumorectomy" followed by chemotherapy. Some groups prefer to perform a biopsy to confirm the diagnosis, give chemotherapy, and then excise the tumors. Currently, study groups are investigating more potent chemotherapy combinations for advanced tumors, and at the same time are attempting to learn what is the minimum amount of chemotherapy necessary for a cure in stage I tumors.

Bibliography

1. Gessler M, Poustka A, Cavenee W, Neve R, Orkin S, Bruns G. Homozygous deletion in Wilms' tumors of a zinc-finger gene identified by chromosome jumping. Nature 1990; 343:774-78.
2. Beckwith J. Wilms' tumors of childhood; a selective review from the NWTS Pathology Center Hum. Pathology 1983; 14:481.
3. Tucker O, McGill C, Pokorny W, et al., Bilateral Wilms' tumors. J Pediat Surg 1986; 21:1110.

21

CHEMOTHERAPY FOR ADVANCED TESTIS CANCER

Merrill Kies, M.D.

Historical Perspective

FOR 25 YEARS, DISSEMINATED testicular cancer has been considered relatively sensitive to cytoxic treatment. Dactinomycin-based regimens produced occasional complete responses (CRs) and probably a 5% cure rate. In the 1960s, combinations of drugs, especially vinblastine (VLB) and bleomycin (BLM), achieved a 10-20% CR rate that proved durable in about half of patients. In the 1970s, the introduction of cisplatin (DDP) heralded a major advance. It is the single most active agent in this disease, and in combination with other active drugs produces CR rates in the range of 80%, the vast majority of which are lasting. Effective tumor markers and improved imaging techniques have defined disease extent and responses more accurately, thereby contributing to improved treatment strategy by better assessment of prognostic factors and more timely identification of refractory disease.

VAB and PVB Programs

DDP-based combination therapy has reliably produced CRs in 50-70% of patients with advanced disease. Of these complete responders, long-term survival is observed in about 80%. The majority of tumor relapses occur within 1 yr of the completion of therapy.

Since the landmark chemotherapy trials of the 1970s, much work has been performed to improve overall treatment efficacy. At Indiana University, the initial PVB regimen was DDP 20 mg/m^2/day x 5, VLB 0.2 mg/kg days 1 and 2, and BLM 30 U/wk. Major toxicity consisted of nausea, constipation and ileus, and myelosuppression. Subsequent studies showed that the VLB dose could be reduced to ameliorate toxicity without sacrifice in tumor response over an induction program of 4 treatment cycles. The Southeastern Cancer Study Group tested the value of maintenance VLB in a prospective, randomized trial and found no advantage. Notably, optimal chemotherapy effects seemed to occur with the initial 12-wk period of therapy. In summary, 202 of 272 patients (74%) treated at Indiana with PVB programs were alive, apparently cured of disseminated testis cancer at a minimum of 8 yr follow-up.

Further work has shown that etoposide (VP-16) can be substituted for VLB with similar therapeutic results and less neurologic toxicity; DDP + VP-16 + BLM has become an accepted front-line regimen for advanced testis cancer.

Staging and Prognostic Factors

The Indiana Staging Schedule is as follows:

Minimal

1. Elevated markers only
2. Cervical ± retroperitoneal nodes
3. Unresectable, nonpalpable retroperitoneal disease
4. Minimal pulmonary metatases: <5 per lung field and largest <2 cm (± nonpalpable abdominal disease; ± cervical nodes)

Moderate

1. Palpable abdominal mass with no supradiagraphmatic disease
2. Moderate pulmonary metastases: 5-10 per lung field with largest < 3 cm; or, solitary pulmonary mass of any size; or, mediastinal adenopathy <50% intrathoracic diameter

Advanced

1. Advanced pulmonary metastases: primary mediastinal germ cell tumor; or, >10 pulmonary metastases per lung field; or, multiple pulmonary metastases with largest metastasis >3 cm
2. Palpable abdominal mass + pulmonary metastases
3. Hepatic, osseous, or CNS metastases

Factors that predict for cure after "appropriate" therapy are histology and tumor volume. Embryonal components predict higher rates of relapse, but tumor bulk and demonstration of adverse patterns of metastases (bone, CNS, liver) most clearly identify the patient with potentially refractory disease. In minimal and moderate disease, a course of 3 cycles (9 wk) of chemotherapy has been found equivalent to 4 cycles, with 5% risk of recurrence on both arms. In advanced disease, ongoing trials are evaluating dose and schedule alterations in comparison to standard DDP combinations. For patients with recurrent cancer, salvage therapy with ifosfamide, DDP, and either VP-16 or VLB may produce durable CRs. Highly intensive therapy with autologous marrow rescue is also an investigational option now under study.

Bibliography

1. Einhorn et al. Cis-diamminedichloroplatinum, vinblastine, and bleomycin combination chemotherapy in disseminated testicular cancer. Ann Intern Med 1977; 87:293-98.
2. Einhorn et al. The role of maintenance therapy in disseminated testicular cancer. N Engl J Med 1981; 305:727-31.
3. Bosl. Treatment of germ cell tumors at Memorial Sloan-Kettering Cancer Center: 1960 to present. In: Garnick MB, ed. Genitourinary cancer: contemporary issues in clinical oncology. vol 5. New York: Churchill Livingstone, 1985; 45.
4. Logothetis et al. Primary chemotherapy for clinical stage II nonseminomatous germ cell tumors of the testis: a follow-up of 50 patients. J Clin Oncol 1987; 5:906-11.
5. Williams et al. Immediate adjuvant chemotherapy versus observation with treatment at relapse in patholocigal stage II testicular cancer. N Engl J Med 1987; 317:1433-8.
6. Loehrer et al. Salvage therapy in recurrent germ cell cancer: ifosfamide and cisplatin plus either vinblastine or etoposide. Ann Intern Med 1988; 109:540-46.
7. Einhorn et al. Evaluation of optimal duration of chemotherapy in favorable-prognosis disseminated germ cell tumors: a Southeastern Cancer Study Group protocol. J Clin Oncol 1989; 7 (3) 387-91.
8. Hesketh et al. Prognostic assessment in nonseminomatous testicular cancer: implications for therapy. J Urol 1990; 144:1-9.
9. Boyer et al. Lack of late toxicity in patients treated with cisplatin-containing combination chemotherapy for metastatic testicular cancer. J Clin Oncol 1990; 8:21-26.

22

TREATMENT OF ADVANCED REFRACTORY TESTIS CANCER WITH AUTOLOGOUS BONE MARROW TRANSPLANTATION

Craig Nichols, M.D.

Introduction

CLINICAL TRIALS IN THE treatment of germ cell cancer have been particularly productive. Development of clinical trials have led to chemotherapy treatments that cure 80% of the patients with disseminated germ cell cancer. Within this framework, important new agents such as cisplatin (DDP), etoposide (VP-16), and ifosfamide (IFX) have become licensed. Of more importance, clinical investigations in germ cell cancer have helped shape and validate general chemotherapy principles such as the importance of intensive induction chemotherapy and the futility of low-dose maintenance treatment.

One alternative to the addition of new drugs to chemotherapy combinations has been attempted dose intensification. Preclinical and clinical studies in germ cell malignancies suggest that this would be a fruitful approach. There is a very steep dose/response curve for DDP in preclinical models, and several clinical trials have suggested improved outcome for patients with germ cell cancer if they receive more DDP-intensive regimens. With the availability of carboplatin (CARB), true dose intensity can be achieved to the 4- to 5-fold range when coupled with autologous bone marrow support. With this background, we developed clinical trials investigating high-dose chemotherapy in refractory testis cancer.

Phase 1-2 Cooperative Trial

Between September 1986 and July 1988, 29 patients with recurrent germ cell cancer at Indiana University were entered on a large phase 1-2 trial in conjunction with Vanderbilt University.[1] Patients were seleced if they had failed initial DDP-containing chemotherapy and a salvage regimen with DDP and IFX or were overtly DDP refractory as defined by progression on DDP or within 4 wk of the last DDP dose. The treatment protocol was designed to deliver 2 consecutive courses of high-dose CARB and VP-16. Only VP-16 and DDP were selected, since the primary anticipated side effect would be myelosuppression. In high doses, CARB has only rarely been associated with oto-, neuro-, or nephrotoxicity. The anticipated myelosuppression could be modulated by the use of autologous bone marrow transplantation.

Eligible patients underwent bone marrow harvest with a target yield of $2x10^8$ mononuclear cells/kg. After harvest, the bone marrow was divided into 2 equal aliquots. CARB and VP-16 were administered on day -7, -5, and -3, followed by infusion of half of the cryopreserved bone marrow on day 0. After hemopoietic recovery, patients were assessed for toxicities and response. Responding patients were given a second course of treatment. VP-16 was given at 400 mg/m^2 every other day for 3 days, and CARB was given in escalating doses beginning at 300 mg/m^2 up to 660 mg/m^2. After determination of the maximally tolerated combination of CARB and VP-16, patients were treated with CARB 500 mg/m^2 and VP-16 400 mg/m^2 on days -7, -5, and -3.

Results of Initial Study

In the initial study, 29 patients were given 49 courses of therapy. Nine patients obtained a complete remission (CR) and 6 obtained a partial remission (PR), for an overall response rate of 52%. Four patients remain in continuous CR at 38+, 36+, 28+, and 24+ mo. In addition, one patient developed a therapy-related myelodysplastic syndrome and died free of germ cell cancer 28 mo after high-dose treatment. Of note, 2 of the long-term survivors were patients who had had progressive disease on DDP therapy.

The primary toxicity of this regimen is myelosuppression. Four patients died during the granulocytopenic nadir. Sepsis contributed to the death of 3 of these patients and veno-occlusive disease plus infection in the fourth patient. Clinically significant enterocolitis was the primary nonhematologic toxicity. Ototoxicity, renal impairment, and neurotoxicity were clinically signifcant complications.

Several similar trials in Europe have demonstrated similar results. At the Institut Gustave Roussy in Lyon, France, Pico, Droz and associates have investigated high-dose therapy with DDP 40 mg/m^2 days 1-5, VP-16 350 mg/m^2 days 1-5, and cyclophosphamide (CTX) 1,600 mg/m^2 days 2-5 (PEC).[2,3] This high-dose therapy was coupled with autologous bone marrow rescue beginning 72 hr after completion of chemotherapy. The preliminary results of this study included 19 patients with recurrent germ cell tumor. Myelosuppression was the only significant toxicity, and extramedullary complications were mild. Two of the 19 patients died from therapy-related causes. Of the 15 patients evaluable for response, 5 remain in continuous CR at 3+ to 51+ mo.

A report from Linkesch et al in Austria combines features of the PET protocol and protocols from Indiana University coupled with hematopoietic growth factors.[4] In this study, high-dose therapy with CARB 2,000 mg/m^2, VP-16 1,500 mg/m^2, and CTX 60 mg/kg x 2 days was given to patients with recurrent and refractory germ cell cancer. Overall, 16 patients were treated with the regimen, including 4 in whom GM-CSF was used to modulate the duration of granulocytopenia. Eight of the 16 patients achieved a PR and 3 patients achieved durable CRs lasting 7+ to 14+ months.

A study similar to the Indiana University study, conducted by Rosti and colleagues in Ravena, Italy, used CARB and VP-16 in the dose and schedule performed at Indiana University.[5] Twenty-one patients entered after failing primary and usually secondary therapy for germ cell cancers. In this patient population, 8 CRs were obtained, with 6 remaining in continuous response at 1+, 2+, 4+, 5+, 5+, and 33+ mo.

Summary

In summary, results from Indiana University and other centers in the United States and Europe suggest that about 20% of patients with recurrent or resistant germ cell cancer can be salvaged with high-dose chemotherapy. The most widely used regimens include CARB and VP-16–based regimens with or without the addition of IFX or CTX. Based on these primary results, investigators have begun to incorporate high-dose chemotherapy into initial salvage therapy or, in some cases, into primary treatment. Indiana University, along with the Eastern Cooperative Oncology Group, is currently beginning an initial salvage program including 2 courses of conventional therapy with vihblastine (VLB), IFX, and DDP, followed by a single round of high-dose CARB and VP-16.

A multicenter French study randomizes poor-risk patients to receive either DDP, VLB, VP-16, and bleomycin alone or the same combination followed by high-dose chemotherapy with DDP, VP-16, and CTX. Memorial Sloan-Kettering Cancer Center has begun a trial of high-dose CARB and VP-16 in patients who have a suboptimal serologic response to conventional initial therapy.

References

1. Nichols CR, Tricot G, Williams SD, et al. Dose-intensive chemotherapy in refractory germ cell cancer—a phase I/II trial of high dose carboplatin and etoposide with autologous bone marrow transplantation. J Clin Oncol 1989; 7:932-39.
2. Pico JL, Ostronoff M, Droz JP, et al. High dose chemotherapy (CT) with cisplatin (CDDP), etoposide (VP-16) and cyclophosphamide (CTX) (PEC Protocol) followed by autologous bone marrow support in nonseminomatous germ cell tumors (NSGCT). Proc Am Soc Clin Oncol 1989; 8:12.
3. Droz JP, Pico JL, Ghosn M, et al. High complete remission (CR) and survival rates in poor prognosis (PP) non-seminomatous germ cell tumors (NSGCT) with high dose chemotherapy (HDCT) and autologous bone marrow transplantation (ABMT). Proc Am Soc Clin Oncol 1989; 8:130.
4. Linkesch W, Kuhrer I, Wagner A. rhu-GM-CSF after ultrahigh dose carboplatin, VP-16, cyclophosphamide with ABMT in refractory germ cell cancer. Proc Am Soc Clin Oncol 1990; 9:141.
5. Rosti G. Personal communication.

23

NEUROBLASTOMA

Susan L. Cohn, M.D.

NEUROBLASTOMA (NB), A MALIGNANT neoplasm of neural crest origin, is one of the most common childhood cancers, comprising 8-10% of the total seen from birth through age 14.[1] Although all NBs are histologically similar (small round blue cells), these tumors have a wide range of clinical virulence. Some NBs progress rapidly despite the administration of intensive chemotherapy and radiotherapy, while others are successfully treated with surgery alone. In addition, NBs occasionally undergo spontaneous regression or maturation to benign ganglioneuroma.[2,3]

Neuroblastoma is also associated with a wide range of clinical presentations. About 70% of the patients present with metastatic disease, and symptoms related to the metastasis, such as bone pain, may be the initial complaint. Patients with large thoracic tumors may have respiratory tract symptoms or symptoms related to superior vena cava obstruction. Neurologic abnormalities secondary to spinal cord compression are not unusual in patients with paraspinal neuroblastomas; these patients require emergency treatment. Babies commonly have subcutaneous nodules secondary to neuroblastoma metastatic to the skin. In addition, patients can have severe diarrhea related to vasoactive intestinal peptide (VIP) excretion from the tumor. The syndrome of opsoclonus and myoclonus is another rare presentation of neuroblastoma.

Numerous clinically important prognostic factors have been identified that help the pediatric oncologist assess patients with NB (table 23-1).[4] The stage of disease and the age of the patient at diagnosis are 2 well-documented prognostic factors. As with other types of cancer, patients with localized tumors have a much better prognosis than those with advanced disease. However, neuroblastoma patients <12 mo

Table 23-1. Neuroblastoma Prognostic Factors

- Stage of disease
- Age at diagnosis
- Serum ferritin
- Serum neuron-specific enolase
- Pattern of urine catecholamine excretion
- Histopathology
- DNA content (ploidy)
- N-myc oncogene copy number
- Presence of 1p deletion

of age at diagnosis have a better outcome than older children with similar stages of disease. The reason for improved survival in infants is unknown.

Although stage and age are extremely helpful in predicting outcome for children with neuroblastoma, additional prognostic factors have been identified that appear to have independent prognostic value. These include tumor markers such as serum ferritin and serum neuron-specific enolase, the pattern of urinary catecholamine excretion, the histopathologic features of the tumor, the DNA content or ploidy of the tumor cells, the karyotype of the tumor and the number of copies of the N-myc oncogene present in the NB.[4,5,6]

In order to fully evaluate the patient with neuroblastoma, the following diagnostic studies should be performed: CBC, bone marrow aspirate and biopsy, coagulation studies, serum ferritin, serum neuron-specific enolase, N-myc and DNA ploidy analysis of tumor tissue, CT (or MRI) of chest and abdomen, bone scan, skeletal survey, and MIBG (meta-iodobenzylguanidine) scan.

The optimal treatment for patients with localized tumors is complete surgical resection. Even patients with postoperative microscopic residual require no adjunctive therapy. The long-term disease-free survival rate for patients with localized disease is well over 90%. The best treatment for patients with more extensive disease remains controversial. Virtually all patients <12 mo of age with hyperdiploid tumors obtain complete durable remissions with 5 courses of chemotherapy consisting of cyclophosphamide and doxorubicin.[5] Unfortunately, infants with diploid and/or N-myc amplified tumors do not respond well to conventional chemotherapy, and more intensive regimens will be needed to improve the outcome of this subset of patients. Similarly, patients 12-24 mo old with hyperdiploid tumors also respond well to 4-drug chemotherapy, whereas those with diploid DNA content and N-myc amplification do poorly.[7] Older children with advanced disease have a <20% long-term survival rate with chemotherapy alone.[7] Trials are currently being conducted using marrow ablative chemotherapy followed by autologous bone marrow transplant, and it appears that this treatment may be curative in some older patients with widely disseminated disease.[8]

To date, enhanced knowledge about the genetic alterations in neuroblastoma has improved our ability to accurately assess the patient with neuroblastoma. It is hoped that further understanding of the biology of NB will lead, in the near future, to much-needed new and innovative therapy for the patient with clinically aggressive NB.

References

1. Young JL, Miller RW. Incidence of malignant tumors in U.S. children. J Pediatr 1975; 86:254-58.
2. Evans A, Gerson J, Schnaufer L. Spontaneous regression of neuroblastoma. Natl Cancer Inst monogr 1976; 44:49-54.
3. Evans AE, D'Angio GJ, Randolph J. A proposed staging for children with neuroblastoma. Cancer 1974; 27:374-78.
4. Evans AE, D'Angio GJ, Propert K, Anderson J, Hann H-W. Prognostic factors in neuroblastoma. Cancer 1987; 59:1853-59.
5. Loot AT, Hayes FA, Nitschke R, McWilliams NB, Green AA. Cellular DNA content as a predictor of response to chemotherapy in infants with unresectable neuroblastoma. N Engl J Med 1984; 311:231-35.
6. Seeger RC, Brodeur GM, Sather H, et al. Association of multiple copies of the N-myc oncogene with rapid progression of neuroblastoma. N Engl J Med 1985; 313:1111-16.
7. Look AT, Hayes FA, Shuster JJ, et al. Clinical relevance of tumor cell ploidy and N-myc gene amplification in childhood neuroblastoma. A Pediatric Oncology Group study. J. Clin Oncol 1991; 9:581-91.
8. August CS, Serota FT, Koch PA, et al. Treatment of advanced neuroblastoma with supralethal chemotherapy, radiation and allogeneic or autologous marrow reconstitution. J Clin Oncol 1984; 2:609-15.

INDEX